INTRODUCTION TO
RADIOLOGIC
TECHNOLOGY

EIGHTH EDITION

WILLIAM J. CALLAWAY, MA, RT(R)
Radiography Educator, Author, Speaker

ELSEVIER

INTRODUCTION TO RADIOLOGIC TECHNOLOGY,
EIGHTH EDITION

ISBN: 978-0-323-64339-9

Notices

Practitioners and researchers must always rely on their own experience and knowledge in evaluating and using any information, methods, compounds or experiments described herein. Because of rapid advances in the medical sciences, in particular, independent verification of diagnoses and drug dosages should be made. To the fullest extent of the law, no responsibility is assumed by Elsevier, authors, editors or contributors for any injury and/or damage to persons or property as a matter of products liability, negligence or otherwise, or from any use or operation of any methods, products, instructions, or ideas contained in the material herein.

Library of Congress Control Number: 2019935087

Content Strategist: Sonya Seigafuse
Content Development Manager: Ellen Wurm-Cutter
Content Development Specialist: Laura Klein
Publishing Services Manager: Deepthi Unni
Project Manager: Janish Ashwin Paul
Design Direction: Maggie Reid

Printed in United States
Last digit is the print number: 9 8 7 6 5 4 3 2 1

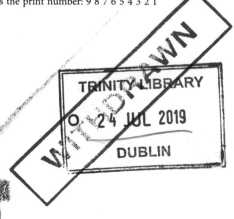
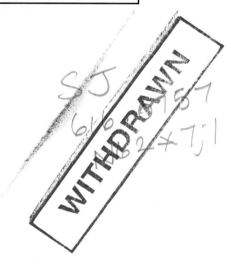
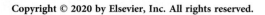

ELSEVIER

3251 Riverport Lane
St. Louis, Missouri 63043

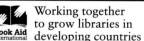
Working together
to grow libraries in
developing countries

www.elsevier.com • www.bookaid.org

INTRODUCTION TO

RADIOLOGIC TECHNOLOGY

I dedicate this new edition to
my best friend and wife, Karen;

our children, Cara, Amy, David, Adam, and Kimberly;

and our grandchildren,
Alex, Kailin, Mariah, Jacob, Mikella, Makenna,
Troy, Madalyn, and Freddy.

A special dedication also goes to Tootsie.

—William J. Callaway

ABOUT THE AUTHOR

William J. Callaway, MA, RT(R), has been involved in radiography education for more than 40 years. He has directed college associate degree and hospital certificate radiography programs. Mr. Callaway is the author of *Mosby's Comprehensive Review of Radiography,* also published by Elsevier, and has published articles in state and national radiologic technology journals. He also co-authored a quality customer service guide for radiology.

He was educated in radiologic technology at Franciscan Medical Center School of Radiologic Technology (now Trinity College of Nursing and Health Sciences) and Black Hawk College in the Illinois Quad-Cities. He earned a bachelor of arts degree from Western Illinois University and a master of arts degree from the University of Illinois.

He has held office in the Association of Collegiate Educators in Radiologic Technology (ACERT) and the Association of Educators in Imaging and Radiologic Sciences (AEIRS). In 2017, he was awarded life membership in ACERT. Mr. Callaway received the Distinguished Alumnus Award from Trinity College of Nursing and Health Sciences and the Dr. LaVerne Gurley award from the Tennessee Society of Radiologic Technologists. He also co-founded Radiography Educators of the Midwest (REM).

Mr. Callaway is widely known for his highly motivational presentations for students, educators, and practicing technologists, which are conducted at national, regional, state, and local radiologic technology conferences. He has presented hundreds of his classes that include "Pass It the First Time: Preparing for the Radiography Certification Exam," "And You Thought X-ray Physics Had to be Boring!," "It's More Than a Smile: A Fresh Perspective on Patient Care," "Win That Job!," "The Key Points of Presenting at Conferences," "Are You Sure You Want to Say It That Way?", and "When You Think You've Seen Everything: The Bizarre Side of Radiology".

PREFACE

CONTENT

This eighth edition of *Introduction to Radiologic Technology* has been reorganized and updated. The hundreds of programs and thousands of students who have used the previous seven editions have confirmed my original belief that a strong introduction and orientation to the profession is vital to a new student who is embarking on a career in radiologic technology. It is gratifying to attend a conference anywhere in the United States and have registered technologists say they began their career with this textbook.

I have, by design, retained the "introductory" nature of this text with the full knowledge that subsequent courses will delve more deeply into the technical aspects of radiography. Chapters have been updated, reorganized, and in some cases merged to remain current with technical advances and changes in the health care system; however, I have taken care, as suggested by readers, to maintain the comprehension level and simple style expected of an introductory course.

The purpose of this new edition remains the same as that of previous editions: to introduce the new or prospective student to the profession of radiologic technology and to the body of knowledge required to become a member of the profession. The intent is to inform students early in their studies of what they can expect from their education, clinical experiences, and patient care, as well as a career in radiologic technology, options for advancement, and what will be required of them. As the health care environment becomes increasingly more challenging, this goal takes on added significance.

NEW TO THIS EDITION

- The sequence of material has been rearranged into a more logical flow. Some chapters have been merged with others to keep related content together in an easier-to-understand context.
- Numerous new photographs and illustrations reflect current equipment and practice.
- End-of-chapter questions are now challenging critical thinking questions and provide for reflection or group interaction and discussion. Previous multiple-choice questions have been moved to the Evolve website.
- Current imaging technology has replaced outdated equipment and procedures.
- Radiation measurement is stated using SI units only.

LEARNING ENHANCEMENTS

Each chapter begins with an outline, key terms, and learning objectives. Chapter content is followed by references and critical thinking style questions that can be used by readers to assess knowledge or by the instructor to encourage discussion. Key terms are shown in **bold** print. These key terms are defined in the chapter and in the glossary that is found in the back of the book.

INSTRUCTOR'S RESOURCES

Instructor's resources are designed to help the instructor encourage active student participation in the class. Instructor's resources, including PowerPoint presentations and multiple-choice questions, are available on the Evolve website at evolve.elsevier.com/

ACKNOWLEDGEMENTS

Deep appreciation goes to the educators and students who, since 1982, have placed this text at the forefront of radiography education. Thousands of radiography students have begun their studies within the pages of this book.

The first seven editions of this text were co-edited with Dr. LaVerne Gurley, PhD, RT(R)(T)(N), with whom I had a unique and productive professional relationship that began with a common dream many years ago. She was credentialed in radiography, radiation therapy, and nuclear medicine and was one of the first radiologic technology educators to earn a PhD. She was truly one of radiologic technology's visionaries. Dr. Gurley researched and authored numerous published articles. She earned countless awards and recognitions for her meritorious service to the profession. She was a fellow and life member of both the American Society of Radiologic Technologists and the Association of Educators in Imaging and Radiologic Sciences. After nearly 30 years with the University of Tennessee medical units, Dr. Gurley transferred to Shelby State Community College in Memphis to direct the radiologic technology program. She retired from full-time service in 1989 and from part-time service in 1996. Her countless friends and colleagues mourned her passing in 2015. It was truly a joy to work with her on this textbook for more than 30 years.

Special recognition goes to all of the previous contributors and reviewers who made the first seven editions so relevant and student friendly. In particular, thanks go to my closest friends and colleagues (you know who you are) who have provided encouragement and motivation as this text became a foundation in radiography programs nationwide.

Thank you to my friends and colleagues Kelli Welch Haynes, EdD, RT(R), at Northwestern State University of Louisiana and Chad Hensley, MEd, RT(R)(MR), at the University of Nevada, Las Vegas, who provided expert critique of my plans for a revised chapter alignment and new table of contents as I began this revision and update. Their enthusiasm for this text was key to making this eighth edition happen.

A sincere note of appreciation goes to Sonya Seigafuse at Elsevier, who guided this new edition through the approval process. Special acknowledgment goes to the all of the professionals at Elsevier who supported this project. This great team of professionals is a joy to work with and is consistently the best at what they do. Special recognition goes to Laura Klein, who guided manuscript development throughout the entire project. Thank you also to Ellen Wurm-Cutter for her leadership of the development team. A very special thank you goes to Janish Paul, with whom I worked on the final stages of this project. His patience and professionalism are very much appreciated. Considering the talents of the entire Elsevier staff, any errors in or omissions from this book are solely mine.

Special recognition goes to my family for their love and support of my many professional involvements, from speaking to writing and all the travel that goes with it. Thanks to my wife Karen; our children Cara, Amy, David, Adam, and Kimberly; and our grandchildren Alex, Kailin, Mariah, Jacob, Mikella, Makenna, Troy, Madalyn, and Freddy. A special recognition goes to Tootsie, who kept me company on my lap or at my feet during my many hours at the computer.

William J. Callaway

CONTENTS

PART I

Becoming a Radiologic Technologist

1

Radiography Education:
From Classroom to Clinic

OBJECTIVES

On completion of this chapter, you should be able to:
- Describe the importance of treating the patient as a guest.
- Discuss the courses essential to the education of radiologic technologists.
- Explain the basic purpose of institutional and programmatic accreditation.
- Explain the relationship between clinical education and the theory component of the radiologic technology curriculum.
- Contrast cognitive, psychomotor, and affective learning.
- Explain what is meant by *clinical competency evaluation.*

KEY TERMS

accreditation
affective learning
clinical competency evaluation
cognitive learning
continuing education
independent clinical performance

institutional accreditation
interaction
maudlin
passive participation
peer review
phantoms

programmatic accreditation
psychomotor learning
radiography curriculum
self-study
site visit
solicitous

WELCOME

Welcome to the study of radiologic technology! You are about to embark on a series of educational experiences designed to help you work in the intriguing and challenging specialty of medical radiography. Whether you are already enrolled in a radiography program or are taking this course as a prerequisite to entering a program, this text will introduce you to the many facets of this profession and the educational process you are now beginning.

Radiography is a specialty within the field of radiologic technology. The professionals working in this field are called radiographers, medical imaging professionals who use x-rays and digital image receptors to acquire diagnostic images.

The Beginning

To provide high-quality service, a thorough understanding of your chosen field is necessary. You must have a command of the technical aspects of radiography so you are free to concentrate on the health care customer, who is traditionally called the *patient*. This book will assist you on your journey. Because education at this level is a complicated task, this chapter and Chapter 2 offer help in understanding the learning process itself. These include ideas and suggestions about how to get started with the study habits and personal adjustments required of a new student, including the information required to establish effective methods of study. Careful attention to this material will help set the stage for all that follows throughout your education in radiography. Lifelong learning is the key to success, and the study habits developed now will serve you well in the years to come.

Part I also presents the history and future of health care in general and of radiology in particular. Although volumes have been written on the history of medicine, Chapter 3 provides a concise treatment of this subject. The history of radiology, in Chapter 4, is particularly interesting and exciting; it is marked by constant change and advances.

The day-to-day practice of radiography is complex. Many new and interesting terms, examinations, and relationships must be learned. Chapters 5 through 9 in Part II introduce patient care, terminology, equipment, examinations, and radiograph production. These topics are immediately encountered on entering the clinical phase of the educational program; therefore they are presented here to begin to give you a working knowledge of what is happening in the radiology department. Your early clinical rotations will mean more to you if you already have a grasp of the imaging environment.

Part II also includes an introduction to patient service as well as discussions on medical ethics and the legal implications of the practice of radiography are presented. These

two areas must be taken seriously throughout the duration of the educational process and beyond to ensure that you practice according to established standards and within legal parameters.

The remainder of Part II deals with topics that you must understand as you work within a radiology department or, as it is called in many institutions, the *imaging department* or *medical imaging*. The operation of a radiology complex is discussed in terms of its organizational structure. Becoming aware of your surroundings enables you to begin to understand your role. Radiology is a very expensive department; hence, you are also introduced to the complex economic issues involved in its operation and maintenance of quality.

Radiologic technologists follow a code of ethics that includes attention to radiation safety and public education. Entering the field of radiography implies that you will accept some exposure to radiation and learn to protect yourself and the public from unnecessary exposure. A complete chapter is devoted to this topic. This knowledge will enable you to feel confident and comfortable as you enter the clinical site, and you will be self-assured as friends, relatives, and patients ask questions about radiation safety. With an understanding of this material, you will be in a position to educate both patients and acquaintances properly.

The entire field of health care has been advancing at a rapid pace. With this rapid advancement has come the increased specialization on the part of physicians and the emergence of many new health care fields (known collectively as the *health professions*). Part II ends with a description of the roles of some of the other members of the health care team who you will encounter during your clinical experiences. Why learn about other health care professionals? The total care of the patient depends on the cooperation and mutual respect of all departments. You will provide services to many of these departments, and other departments will provide services to radiology. All departments exist to provide high-quality service to patients, families, and physicians. Teamwork requires that everyone understands the role of the other members. In this treatment of the subject, you will learn about the educational background and job responsibilities of the fellow professionals you will encounter during patient care. You will soon realize that everyone is equally important in providing clinical care and service to the sick or injured.

Part III addresses the professional aspects of radiologic technology. Serious, career-minded professionals need to know as much as possible about the field and the opportunities it provides. The American Registry of Radiologic Technologists (ARRT) is discussed, and its role as the certifying agency for thousands of radiologic technologists is explained. Professional organizations, all dedicated to providing members the finest in continuing education and professional representation, are also described. These organizations play an important role in your education, as well as in your career plans.

Part III also discusses career advancement and clinical specialization in radiologic technology. A career in this profession can take you in many directions. Although you are only beginning your career, this discussion will help you better understand the varied opportunities available in this field; it is never too early to begin setting long-term goals.

Again, congratulations on being accepted to study in the field of health care! In few other careers can you find the potential for doing so much good while achieving satisfaction. Your future studies will be interesting and intriguing as you strive to become a professional in your field. As you study and observe those around you, you will come to know what is meant by the term *professional*. You will see both positive and negative examples of professional performance; before long, you will be able to decide which of these you want to emulate in your daily work. The title *professional* is earned through dedication and hard work; you cannot purchase it with tuition dollars. As you progress in your studies, take pride in what you do and act appropriately. Your growth as a professional does not end when you become a radiographer; it will continue throughout your career. You must act like a professional and demand to be treated like one, and you must also remember that you, as well as all other health care workers, are important to the patient's well-being.

During the next 2 to 4 years, you will have the chance to examine your career goals and personal expectations. Enjoy your studies and your chosen profession. Although much hard work is involved, it can be satisfying. Make the most of this time, and you will construct a secure foundation for a lifetime career in professional health care. Remember, mastering the technical portions of medical radiography will free you to concentrate on the reason you came into this field—to provide people with the best care you can.

To the novice, the work performed by a well-educated registered technologist may seem methodic, repetitious, and lacking challenge. However, on close examination, it becomes apparent that the technologist must possess complex knowledge and apply it to the radiologic examination of patients.

The reason a particular occupation or task appears easy is that the person performing the job has learned the many intricacies involved. This statement is particularly true with radiologic technology. The educated technologist provides every patient with optimal patient care, which includes interaction with the patient, positioning, procedures, and the selection of exposure factors that produce the best diagnostic radiologic examination. Therefore, the performance of various tasks might appear easy to the patients and others outside the profession.

THE PATIENT AS OUR GUEST

As you contemplate the beginning of your studies, it is crucial to understand the key individual in the health care setting is the patient. This means that we must think of the patient as our guest. Examining this phrase and understanding how the patient is a guest is very important. The patient is the recipient of the many services provided in medical facilities. On admission to the hospital, clinic, or physician's office, the patient is abruptly introduced to an unusual environment filled with wondrous, unnamed machines and a variety of people, all waiting for the guest—the patient.

When a qualified physician requests a radiographic examination, it becomes the radiographer's responsibility to:
1. Interact with the patient.
2. Establish and maintain an atmosphere of caring and empathy for the patient.
3. Treat the patient as a guest in a home.

Essentially, this treatment should be respectful without being familiar, empathetic without being **maudlin** (tearful, emotional), considerate without being **solicitous** (fearful, overly concerned), and professional without being cold and clinical.

This all sounds like a tall order, especially when the workload is heavy, the hour grows late, and more things are yet to be done, but you only need to put yourself in the place of the patient to understand the importance of a health care professional's responsibility (Fig. 1.1).

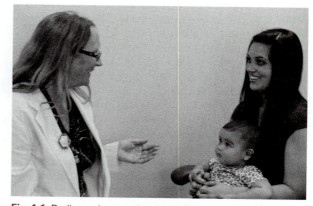

Fig. 1.1 Radiographer treating the patient as a guest and gaining trust by explaining the procedure. (From Lampignano JP, Kendrick LE: *Bontrager's handbook of radiographic positioning and techniques*, ed 9, St. Louis, 2018, Elsevier.)

When caring for very young or very old patients, terminally ill patients, or patients with disabilities, this responsibility may be difficult to handle. These patients do not, however, change the importance of these responsibilities. This responsibility is the basis of being in a helping profession. Above all, every patient who comes to radiology is a guest! We will discuss providing quality patient service in Chapter 6.

This chapter introduces students to the work of a radiologic technologist, provides the minimum core curriculum necessary for entry-level performance, and discusses evaluations you will encounter during the learning process.

ACCREDITATION

Accreditation is a process of external quality control. Through a process of **peer review**, a nongovernmental agency attests to the adequacy of an institution or program in meeting established standards. Students enrolled in a program of study in the radiologic sciences will likely encounter accreditation in several ways: the educational program in which they are enrolled may be accredited, the educational institution that sponsors the educational program may be accredited, and the clinical settings where they receive clinical education and experience may be housed in accredited institutions.

Two forms of educational accreditation have been established: institutional and specialized. **Institutional accreditation** seeks to assess the overall quality and integrity of an institution. Most colleges that sponsor radiologic sciences programs are accredited by one of several regional or national (institutional) accrediting agencies. Specialized accreditation, or **programmatic accreditation**, on the other hand, seeks to address educational endeavors at the program level. The Joint Review Committee on Education in Radiologic Technology (JRCERT) is approved to evaluate the quality and integrity of individual radiologic technology programs. In addition, most health care institutions (hospitals and clinics) are accredited by The Joint Commission (TJC). In the broadest sense, accreditation exists to safeguard the public.

At the program level, particularly in the health fields, the adequacy of education is of significant concern to the general public. The accreditation of programs in radiologic sciences that voluntarily meet standards establishes that these programs adhere to nationally developed professional education standards in their preparation of these health care professionals. It assures the public, the profession, and the students who graduate are adequately prepared for professional practice as determined by the profession. Program accreditation authorities review and evaluate criteria more directly related to the profession, such as the curriculum, specific faculty qualifications, and clinical experience and supervision. Even programs that are not programmatically accredited often follow most of the same standards as accredited programs. Both institutional and programmatic accreditation are acceptable to the ARRT for students applying to take the national certification examination.

Particularly in the case of radiologic technology, attention is paid to radiation safety issues and student supervision to ensure quality patient care. From the earliest days after Roentgen's discovery of the x-ray in 1895, the need for proper training in the use of this powerful force was recognized. The first physicians who experimented with the use of the Roentgen ray in the diagnosis of disease informally trained x-ray "technicians" on an as-needed basis. The onset of more formal training programs began with radiologists and technicians working together to establish instructional programs in a few hospitals. The American Medical Association (AMA) was recognized as the official accrediting agency at one time. Today the JRCERT accredits more than 700 radiography, radiation therapy, medical dosimetry, and magnetic resonance educational programs along with recognizing more than 7000 clinical education settings as affiliates for educational programs in the radiologic sciences.

Standards

The standards that an educational program are required to meet to achieve and maintain accreditation are developed over time through consensus building involving the entire profession. The results are discussed in the JRCERT document *Standards for an Accredited Educational Program Radiography*, as well as similar documents for other specialties in radiologic technology. These standards all define requirements in the areas of mission and goals, program integrity, organization, and administration, curriculum, resources, students, safety, and program assessment and effectiveness.

Students should be aware of the accreditation standards their programs are required to meet if it has programmatic accreditation. Many educational programs provide a copy of the accreditation standards in their student handbooks or post them on a bulletin board that is accessible to the student body. Students can also access this information by visiting the JRCERT website (www.jrcert.org) or by contacting the JRCERT office.

Maintenance of Accreditation

Accredited programs must comply with requirements for maintaining accreditation. Such requirements involve the faculty writing a report of **self-study**, undergoing an on-site visit from the JRCERT, maintaining adherence to the accreditation standards, and writing an interim report of accreditation half-way through the accreditation period, which normally extends 8 years. If you are enrolled in an accredited program at the time of a **site visit**, you and your classmates will be interviewed by the site visitors regarding your experiences in the program.

Failure to comply with established requirements will result in the program being placed on probation. The JRCERT is required by the United States Department of Education (USDE) to be responsive to allegations that an accredited program is not in compliance with educational standards. A summary of the allegations and the program's response is presented to the JRCERT Board of Directors for consideration and action. After deliberation, the board may decide that the allegations are without merit, that the allegations are true but that the program has taken appropriate action, or that the program is in noncompliance with one or more of the educational standards.

Value of JRCERT Accreditation

The impact of accreditation is diverse, given that it affects students, institutions, and society in general. In its broadest sense, accreditation ensures acceptable educational quality as defined by the profession.

Perhaps the most significant benefit of JRCERT accreditation is assurance to the public that graduates have met the minimal level of competency as defined nationally by the profession. It also assures the public, through radiation safety and supervision standards, that students who perform procedures are meeting established professional standards.

The process of peer review assures students who graduate from an accredited program that they have the knowledge, skills, and values to perform competently and to meet the expectations of employers nationwide. Some state licensing boards require graduation from a JRCERT-accredited program in addition to certification by the national credentialing agency.

Some employers, as well, require graduation from a JRCERT-accredited program. Thus graduation from a JRCERT-accredited program makes students more marketable and assists in ensuring mobility of practice because the graduates have met national standards. By hiring graduates of an accredited program, employers are also assured that their personnel have met national professional standards.

The process of accreditation, including an external peer assessment of program quality, contributes to the continuing improvement of an educational program. Through the process of self-evaluation required by the self-study process and the on-site review by peers of the program and its operations, the educational program must continue to evaluate and evolve to become better and stronger.

The JRCERT is the organization with the primary function of documenting the compliance of educational programs in the radiologic sciences with the standards that have been established by the radiologic sciences profession. The process for programmatic accreditation is rigorous but well defined and organized and serves to assure the public and the profession that accredited programs meet the profession's minimal standards for quality. The contact information for the JRCERT is:

Joint Review Committee on Education in Radiologic
   Technology
20 North Wacker Drive, Suite 2850
Chicago, IL 60606-3182
www.jrcert.org

YOUR RESPONSIBILITIES IN HEALTH CARE

No substitute exists for the knowledge necessary to perform the tasks of a radiologic technologist with confidence, effectiveness, and efficiency.

This confidence is a direct result of being prepared. Students are confronted with quizzes, competency tests, and finally, the certifying examination. Yet the greatest tests will come with every radiologic examination you perform. Educators in radiologic technology are aware of the need for well-prepared radiologic technologists.

The field of radiology is continually changing and has accelerated in the wake of space age technology. However, learning the basic principles of the production of x-radiation and how to make these principles work is imperative for student radiologic technologists.

What does a radiologic technologist need to know to perform the responsibilities of radiologic technology? To answer this question, you need to look at the course recommendations for programs in radiologic technology, as well as the unique goals and needs of the sponsoring institutions and clinical affiliates.

THE RADIOGRAPHY CURRICULUM

Radiography programs follow the national **radiography curriculum** written by educators and technologists on the curriculum revision committee of the American Society of Radiologic Technologists (ASRT). The draft curriculum document is then published for the entire profession to comment on, and ultimately, approve. It is a curriculum that is created and supported by the entire profession.

There is much to learn in your program, as evidenced by typical course offerings covering: patient care, anatomy and physiology and pathology, radiographic positioning and procedures, imaging technology, radiation biology and protection, x-ray production, image acquisition and evaluation, venipuncture, medical ethics and legal issues, and, of course, clinical education. Clinical education will make up a large portion of your studies. Your program may also include introductions to computed tomography and sectional anatomy.

Actual course titles will vary by program but will include all of these subjects. Some courses may combine topics, but the entire curriculum will be covered. These courses are all in addition to the specific requirements for your associate or baccalaureate degree. Typical radiography courses are summarized next.

Introduction to Radiography

This course is designed to introduce students to the basic aspects of the department of imaging, radiologic technology, and the health care system in general. The basic principles of radiation protection are introduced. Students should gain a better understanding of the structure and function of agencies through which medical services are delivered.

Clinical Education

Sometimes also called "clinical internship," this course places the student in a clinical setting in order to practice patient care, radiographic positioning, and participation in radiographic procedures. This is where students have the opportunity to demonstrate mastery of knowledge and skills learned in the classroom and lab. Working alongside registered radiographers, students will, over the course of several semesters, assume a steadily increasing role in the performance of medical radiography. This course includes clinical competency and affective behavior evaluations. Most clinical sites use this time to evaluate students for possible hire upon graduation.

Medical Ethics and Law

What are the moral, legal, and professional responsibilities of a radiologic technologist? This course helps students understand how to deal with confidential information and the interpersonal relationships, or **interaction**, with patients and other health care team members. In addition, attention is given to medicolegal considerations, as well as to professional guidelines and codes of ethics.

Principles of Diagnostic Imaging

This course introduces students to digital image acquisition. These images result from the fluoroscopic and radiographic application of the principles of image production. Students are expected to comprehend and apply the principles in the lab and clinical settings.

Imaging Equipment

This course describes the x-ray circuit, x-ray tube, and the process of x-ray production.

Human Structure and Function

This course refers to the anatomy and physiology of the human body. For a radiologic technologist to conduct radiologic procedures on various anatomic parts, knowing the location and function of all body parts is necessary.

Medical Terminology

The written and spoken language of medicine incorporates many uncommon words, meanings, and symbols. For a radiologic technologist to work effectively in radiology, understanding the language of medicine is also necessary.

Radiographic Positioning and Procedures

Every radiology department has a routine for performing procedures specific to that particular department. These procedures range from normal radiographic imaging to more complex tasks requiring contrast media, special radiographic equipment, and accessory materials.

Principles of Radiation Biology and Radiation Protection

The technologist must know how to use ionizing radiation in a safe and prudent manner. Patients, as well as radiologic technologists and coworkers, must be protected from radiation as much as possible. Therefore radiologic technologists must know how exposure factors affect radiation doses, the effective dose limits, and the methods for monitoring exposure. The objective is to practice the *as low as reasonably achievable* (ALARA) concept in diagnostic radiography.

Radiographic Image Evaluation

What is the difference between an optimal quality image and a nondiagnostic one (Fig. 1.2)? This course integrates all of the material previously learned. Although radiographers do not interpret radiographs, they evaluate them for diagnostic quality, which includes the consideration of pathologic conditions.

Pathology

Students need to be acquainted with the various disease conditions that may affect the resulting radiographic images. In addition, knowledge of disease entities is helpful in working with patients.

Patient Care

Through information presented in this course, the radiographer prepares to work with patients, regardless of their

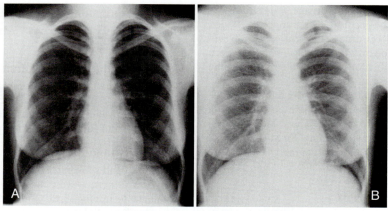

Fig. 1.2 **A,** Optimal-quality radiograph. **B,** Nondiagnostic radiograph.

health conditions, in a manner that does not cause them additional injury or discomfort or hinder their recovery.

Quality Assurance

Optimal quality radiographs achieve many important benefits. They (1) minimize the patient's exposure to radiation, (2) provide the physician with the best possible image for diagnosis, and (3) contain health care costs. Students must know the regulations that govern quality assurance, as well as the techniques, equipment, and procedures for attaining it.

FROM THE CLASSROOM TO THE CLINICAL SETTING

During classroom preparation, students may practice taking radiographs in the lab using **phantoms**, whose x-ray attenuation and scattering properties are similar to those of body tissues. This helps students to learn proper anatomic positioning and exposure techniques. Lab competency exams also take place using classmates as patients and an evaluation form provided by your program. Every detail of an exam will take place except for making an x-ray exposure. One or more of your instructors will observe and score you on your performance. These are stressful demonstrations of your skills that must be passed before being approved to perform each exam in clinical.

After classroom and lab preparation, clinical experience offers the opportunity for student radiographers to perform actual radiographic examinations on real patients. Patients with differing health problems are encountered, hundreds of procedures are experienced, and rules of behavior and ethics by which to abide are learned. In the clinical experience situation, students have the opportunity to prove their understanding of the classroom material by competently performing various radiologic procedures.

CLINICAL PARTICIPATION

Clinical participation is the integration of the cognitive, affective, and psychomotor aspects of radiologic technology education.

Cognitive learning refers to classroom lectures and demonstrations of theories, as well as to the facts and background information necessary to understand a specific body of knowledge. After this fundamental information has been learned, the student has the opportunity to participate in the clinical setting, where each student has the opportunity to apply the knowledge gained from the classroom setting.

Affective learning involves attitudes, values, and feelings. The clinical environment provides the opportunity to develop pride in your work, as well as feelings of self-worth; skills in interpersonal relationships; and personal, moral, and ethical beliefs for daily practice.

Psychomotor learning is the actual hands-on phase—the application of previously learned material. Didactic information is put to actual use in the clinical situation.

The student participates as follows:

1. Assists the practicing radiologic technologist and observes each detail of the radiographic procedure. This involvement is considered **passive participation** because the student is observing.
2. Performs various assigned tasks associated with procedures after becoming familiar with them. The performance of any task depends on the student's ability to understand the responsibilities involved with the assigned tasks and to perform these tasks correctly.
3. Progresses into the **independent clinical performance** phase. This involvement means that the student will perform all aspects of the procedure with appropriate supervision of a registered technologist.

During this time, the student's learning ability and performance are evaluated. The student now has the opportunity to demonstrate knowledge of the subject material and how well each task can be accomplished.

As the student makes the transition from a classroom environment to one that combines both classroom and clinical experience, the learning process becomes integrated and more complex. The student is expected to be more aware of the responsibilities in learning. This means the student must answer the following questions:

1. What do I know?
2. What must I learn?
3. How well have I learned the basic material?
4. Can I apply the classroom information in the clinical setting?

During this phase of radiography education, the student also learns the importance of meeting the objectives of the educational process. Because competency levels vary from individual to individual, these objectives are self-paced. However, a great deal of coordination exists between classroom learning and clinical application. This coordination is facilitated by the program director, working as a team with the clinical coordinator and clinical instructors. These individuals plan the course work and clinical participation that provide an optimal learning environment for the students (Box 1.1).

CLINICAL COMPETENCY EVALUATION

The competency skills of a student radiographer in the clinical setting are evaluated using a clinical competency evaluation. Most likely you will have to perform an examination several times before attempting a clinical competency. The program will provide you with a copy of the form, which will be similar to the one used to evaluate competency in

---

BOX 1.1 Sample Clinical Education Checklist

Orientation to Room

1. Become familiar with the full operation of the x-ray table (tilt, floating tabletop, raising and lowering features, footboard, operation of the Bucky tray).
2. Become familiar with the full operation of the x-ray tube (longitudinal, vertical, transverse, collimator).
3. In fluoroscopic rooms, become familiar with image intensifier, either tube or flat panel.
4. Become familiar with x-ray control panel (setting exposure technique manually or using anatomically programmed radiography, fluoroscopic timer, Bucky selection, automatic exposure control [AEC], on-off switch, performance of warm-up procedure).
5. Be aware of all types of procedures that are performed in the room.
6. Locate all appropriate supplies in the room.
7. Become familiar with the full operation of the wall Bucky.
8. If contrast media are used for any procedures in the room, become familiar with their preparation.

Tasks To Be Performed

1. Set up the room for each procedure before the patient is brought into the room.
2. Assist with or perform all imaging procedures in the assigned room.
3. If it is necessary to consult your notes, do so before you bring the patient into the room. At no time let the patient see you consulting your notes.
4. You are an adult pursuing a new career. Take charge to the best of your ability. If in doubt, ask the registered technologist all questions but not in front of the patient.

5. Courtesy is essential when providing service to the patient during the greeting, procedure, and dismissal phases of the examination.
6. Position the patient professionally and confidently. Position the part to be radiographed, adjust it, and make the exposure.
7. Initially, you may have to ask the radiographer with whom you are working how to set exposure technique.
8. After completing the procedure and dismissing the patient, critique the images with the radiographer. You should be able to identify all pertinent anatomy.
9. Immediately prepare the room for the next patient.

Things to Do with Free Time During Clinical Hours

1. Stock additional supplies wherever necessary.
2. Clean x-ray tabletop, footstool, control panel, wall Bucky, and any other equipment used.
3. Practice positioning using a radiologic technologist as the patient.
4. Go through your notes and review positioning and centering points.
5. Check to see what other procedures are scheduled for that room later in the day and familiarize yourself with them so you can take the initiative in performing them.
6. Clinical hours are for clinical education. Textbook studying generally should not occur during this time. However, during slow periods or equipment breakdown in your assigned area, studying is expected.

BOX 1.2   Sample Clinical Competency Form

Radiography Program
Radiographic Exam Competency Form

Student_____Date_____

Exam_____Practice:_____Practice:_____

Room_____Medical Records Number_____

Number of Images Sent_____ Pt. History_____

Yes No Student passed this competency exam.

Radiographer Signature: _____Date_____

If yes, your signature verifies that all of the above information is accurate. You are confident that this student may now perform this exam with minimal supervision. If no, please indicate difficulties the student encountered: _____

_____

Yes No Student informed the radiographer this was a competency test PRIOR to start.

Yes No Student verified order per clinical site protocol for inpatient or outpatient.

Yes No Date of birth, patient name, and exam were verified with the patient.

Yes No Student introduced self to the patient.

Yes No Student washed hands or used sanitizer in front of patient.

Yes No History was obtained.

Yes No Shielding / Collimation / Markers visible / All radiation safety was appropriate.

Yes No Student set own technique.

Yes No Positioning was accurate.

Yes No There were, or would have been, repeat exposures.

If Yes, why and which projection(s)?_____

Where was the radiographer during the exam? Control panel in the room

Explain any assistance provided by the radiographer_____

Circle one: Table Bucky Upright Bucky Tabletop Portable Surgery

Projection: _____ mAs_____ kVp _____ Exposure Index: _____

Projection: _____ mAs_____ kVp _____ Exposure Index: _____

Projection: _____ mAs_____ kVp _____ Exposure Index: _____

Projection: _____ mAs_____ kVp _____ Exposure Index: _____

Projection: _____ mAs_____ kVp _____ Exposure Index: _____

Projection: _____ mAs_____ kVp _____ Exposure Index: _____

Student:

Yes No I have issues or concerns that I experienced regarding this exam that I would like to discuss.

Yes No I would like to meet to go over items related to this exam, e.g., positioning, technique, etc.

If you did not pass this competency, what could you have done differently? _____

_____

Student Signature:_____Date_____

Your signature verifies that all of the above information is accurate. We may verify any of the above information with the radiographer.

---

the radiography skills lab (Box 1.2). This evaluation is designed to be a positive experience. It is an opportunity for students to gain confidence by becoming thoroughly familiar with each detail of the assigned tasks.

Simply defined, **clinical competency evaluation** is a method of standardizing the evaluation of a student radiographer's performance in the clinical setting. The student must fully appreciate and understand the importance of a standard evaluation concept and its methodology. Typically, the three specific aspects of learning are addressed in this evaluation of performance: cognitive, affective, and psychomotor.

Examinations vary in emphasis, depending on the teaching institution. However, the final objective is always that each student be able to perform all examinations successfully, regardless of specific emphasis, because routines for procedures vary from institution to institution. The ARRT, the organization certifying radiologic technologists, determines clinical competency requirements for programs, although most programs exceed such requirements. Upon completion of the program, your program director must verify that the didactic and clinical skills have been satisfied. Therefore you may expect frequent testing and evaluation throughout your course of study.

CONTINUING EDUCATION AND CONTINUING QUALIFICATIONS REQUIREMENT

The ARRT requires **continuing education** for all ARRT registrants. Each ARRT registrant must obtain either 24 continuing education credits acceptable to ARRT every 2 years or pass an examination in an additional discipline. Furthermore, every 10 years, each technologist must perform a self-assessment and determine if focused continuing education credits are needed to remain current in the profession. These requirements are discussed in Chapter 14.

CONCLUSION

Educators in radiologic technology are aware that for student radiographers, the transition from classroom to clinic can be not only demanding but also, at times, confusing. Programs make every effort to ensure that students are better prepared to accept and deal with this transition. In addition, educators work to ensure that each student is evaluated on a fair and objective basis according to acceptable standards and institutional requirements for the completion of the program.

From time to time, changes are made in the current procedures as new ideas and developments occur in radiologic technology. These changes are incorporated into the curriculum to ensure that students are familiar with new concepts and procedures.

No substitute exists for being well prepared to practice your chosen profession. For students, this time must be spent preparing for the challenges presented with each radiologic procedure. Each radiologic procedure is, after all, a test of your ability to perform the assigned tasks in an efficient, cheerful, and professional manner.

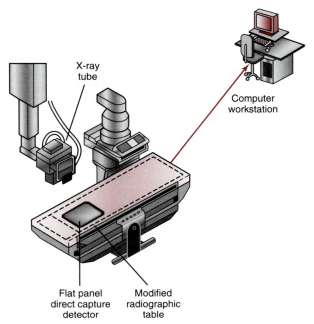

X-ray tube

Computer workstation

Flat panel direct capture detector

Modified radiographic table

Fig. 1.3 Typical digital image acquisition equipment. (From Fauber TL: *Radiographic imaging and exposure*, ed 5, St. Louis, 2017, Elsevier).

It is imperative that each student consider education in radiologic technology as a continuing process. These courses are an indication of the important responsibilities of every radiologic technologist. This material must be learned and understood before you can correctly and safely operate the complicated equipment (Fig 1.3). You need to know not only how the equipment works but also why it works as it does. You must also be able to provide the physician with the best diagnostic radiographic study possible regardless of the patient's condition.

Look closely at each task as it is encountered and study not only the work involved but also the concepts behind the tasks. You should not be surprised to learn that radiologic technology education must be an ongoing process.

QUESTIONS FOR DISCUSSION AND CRITICAL THINKING

1. Explain the importance of treating each patient as a guest in the imaging department.
2. Discuss the major areas of study in a radiography program, describing those you think may be difficult.
3. Compare programmatic accreditation with institutional accreditation.
4. Describe the purpose of lab and clinical competency evaluations and discuss why they may be stressful.
5. Describe cognitive, affective, and psychomotor learning as they pertain to learning radiography.
6. Discuss the importance of staying busy in clinical education.

BIBLIOGRAPHY

American Registry of Radiologic Technologists. *Primary eligibility pathway handbook*. St. Paul, MN: The Registry; 2019.

Fauber T. *Radiographic imaging and exposure*. ed 5. St. Louis: Elsevier; 2017.

Harris EL, Young P, McElveny C, et al. *The shadowmakers: a history of radiologic technology*. Albuquerque, NM: American Society of Radiologic Technologists; 1995.

Joint Review Committee on Education in Radiologic Technology. *Standards for an accredited educational program in radiography*. Chicago: Joint Review Committee on Education in Radiologic Technology; 2014.

2

Becoming an Outstanding Student

OBJECTIVES

On completion of this chapter, you should be able to:
- Identify the needs common to all individuals.
- Describe physiologic needs and their effect on learning.
- Describe the way you perceive the world and your unique pattern of behavior for satisfying your needs.
- Examine your lifestyle to identify causes of stress and conflict.
- Examine your values and determine what is and what is not important to you.
- Describe ways in which conflict may be resolved.
- Increase your skills in memory and recall.
- Explain how perception is influenced by your memory of sights, sounds, and events.
- Improve your listening skills and reading effectiveness.
- Examine inaccurate memory and distortions in remembering and explain the theories for why these inaccuracies occur.
- Identify the qualities of a critical thinker.
- Identify the assumptions, ethics, and values in written works.
- Discern fallacies in arguments.
- Control psychological impediments to sound reasoning.
- Recognize the effects of authors' background beliefs on reasoning.
- Present valid facts, evidence, and statistics.

OUTLINE

Knowing Your Human Needs
  First Level
  Second Level
  Third Level
  Fourth Level
  Fifth Level
Physiologic Needs
  Nutrition
  Sleep
  Recreation and Exercise
Psychologic Needs
  Emotionality
  Objectivity
Emotional and Primal Stress
Stress and Conflict
  Stress
  Conflict
  Managing and Resolving Conflict
Learning how to Learn
Intentional Memorization
  Perception
  Attention

  Improving Listening Skills
  Improving Reading Skills
Retrieving From Memory
Forgetting
  Forgetting: Pain, Pleasure
  Errors in Remembering
  Understanding Critical Thinking
Need for Critical Thinking
  What Is Critical Thinking?
  Qualities of a Critical Thinker
Factors That Hinder Critical Thinking
  Background Beliefs
  Faulty Reasoning
  Group Loyalty
  Frozen Mind-Set
  Emotional Baggage
Becoming a Critical Thinker
  Humility
  Respect for Others
  Self-Awareness
  Honing Your Skills
Conclusion

KEY TERMS

attention
conflict
controlled environment
critical thinking
emancipation
emancipatory learning
emotionality
herd instinct

hierarchy of human needs
long-term memory
memory retrieval
memory storage
objectivity
perceptions
personality
primal stress

psychologic care
reinforcement behavior
rote memorization
self-discipline
short-term memory
stress

Choosing a vocation is an explicit statement about the kind of person you are or hope to be. Professional satisfaction will depend on the extent to which you can use your abilities in a productive manner. Your work should be consistent with your values and interests and the roles you fulfill in society. Choosing radiologic technology is an exploration. Education in radiologic technology is vastly different from the learning acquired in high school or a liberal arts college; the main difference is that your curriculum will require you to spend much of your time in the clinical setting, where you will learn how to manage sick and injured patients. Because patient care is the focus of your curriculum, generally the code of conduct is more rigidly defined and is based on the moral and ethical standards associated with the medical profession. You should expect and understand these differences to avoid future frustration or disappointment.

All students experience some frustration, anxiety, and perhaps a degree of disillusionment in preparing for their careers. Fortunately, most students adjust to these irritants with only minor strain. This chapter is provided to help you cope with the rigors of your educational program by learning about yourself and learning how to learn.

KNOWING YOUR HUMAN NEEDS

Knowing yourself is the most important information you can possess at the beginning of your education. You have your own unique pattern of solving problems and your own values, ambitions, aspirations, and experiences in addition to the basic needs common to everyone; these qualities make up your unique **personality**. Indeed, personality is a combination of habitual patterns and qualities of behavior and attitudes. You think, feel, and act according to your perceptions of the world. You are a seeker, and your thoughts, feelings, and actions are purposefully directed toward satisfying your needs.

Human needs are complex. Some are unique to the individual, and others are common to everyone. Abraham H.

Maslow, a noted psychologist, described a **hierarchy of human needs** that ranges from basic needs that are essential to life (e.g., food, clothing, shelter) to the highly complex, psychologic, and self-actualization needs (Fig. 2.1). Maslow's hierarchy of needs is listed in the following order:

First Level

Needs that are essential to life are first in the order of importance. These needs are food, clothing, shelter, and the will to reproduce.

Second Level

A feeling of safety is essential to growing and developing. You can never be completely safe from physical injury or disease. Feeling a degree of safety in your social and physical environment, however, is important.

Third Level

The need to be loved is inherent. You need the emotional support of others and the warmth and closeness of those important to you. This need also includes the desire to love others, to return affection, and to support and care for those who love you.

Fourth Level

You also need satisfying relationships with others in the larger social community. You need to be valued, accepted, and appreciated to maintain self-esteem, self-respect, and a unique identity.

Fifth Level

Creativity, self-expression, and achievement are also needs characteristic of all human beings. Work needs to be useful, productive, and valuable to others.

The higher-level needs are not felt until the first-level needs are satisfied. For example, a drowning man gasping for air does not feel the need to be creative at that moment. A person with extreme hunger and thirst feels the need for

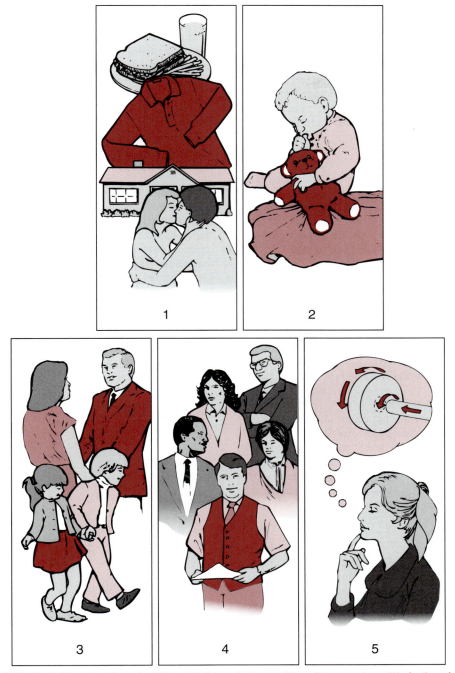

Fig. 2.1 Maslow's hierarchy of needs: *(1)* food, clothing, shelter, and the will to reproduce; *(2)* a feeling of safety; *(3)* love; *(4)* satisfying relationships; and *(5)* creativity, self-expression, and achievement.

love and affection less than the more immediate and urgent need for sustenance. Physical needs must be met before creativity and other higher-level needs are felt.

PHYSIOLOGIC NEEDS

Optimal health and well-being require attention to nutrition, sleep, relaxation, and exercise. To expect optimal learning performance, you must take optimal care of your body.

Nutrition

Diet, nutrition, and learning are tightly interwoven. Learning is easier with a sound body, and a sound body can help produce a sound mind. Nutritional biochemicals keep body cells healthy and functioning, and these biochemicals come from only one source—what you eat. An improper diet can also result in unexplained emotional upsets such as crying, depression, and even violent impulses.

Sleep

Your body also requires adequate sleep, which offers rest to the brain and nervous system. In preparing for your career, you should be relaxed and well rested when you enter the classroom and laboratory so that you and your body can easily meet the demands placed on you. Both sleep and adequate diet are crucial to the learning process.

Recreation and Exercise

Recreation and exercise are important for both the mind and the body. Use of the mind can tire an individual. The mind functions better when mental concentration alternates with periods of diversion and exercise. Proper diet, rest, and recreation are valuable ways to practice personal preventive health care and are essential tools for creating optimal learning conditions.

PSYCHOLOGIC NEEDS

Psychologic care involves developing and maintaining a healthy balance between rational thoughts and emotions. Although your studies will require a great deal of self-discipline, maintaining healthy social interactions with family and friends and accepting your emotions as a natural part of your personality are also important.

Emotionality

Emotionality is the quality or state of a sound emotional balance. Living by values based on a healthy balance between mind and heart and maintaining a sound emotional balance can help you decide what is and what is not important and can help enhance your learning.

Objectivity

Objectivity is the quality or state of being objective, that is, the ability to interpret a situation from an unbiased point of view rather than from your own subjective view. Learning to use rational thought in making decisions will enhance your objectivity. You will learn more about this later in this chapter. Learning to be objective about your behavior, as well as that of others, will help you become a mentally and emotionally healthy person.

EMOTIONAL AND PRIMAL STRESS

You seldom encounter the stress of a life-threatening event as did the early cave dwellers, but your body responds to stress in the same way (Fig. 2.2). Imagine being stalked by a hungry predator. Your heartbeat accelerates, your blood pressure rises, and hormones rush into your bloodstream to send sugar to your muscles and brain. Food digestion temporarily ceases so that more blood is available for energy. In this way, your body prepares to fight the beast or flee to safety. This type of acute stress, which requires a fight-or-flight response, is what McQuade and Aikman call the first primal stress. Because the body does not identify the source of the fear, it reacts in the same way when you get what is commonly known as "stage fright." Stage fright is not life threatening, but for some, the fear they experience

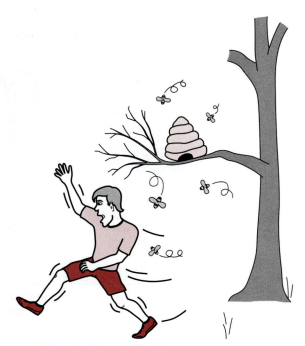

Fig. 2.2 Flight, the body's response to danger.

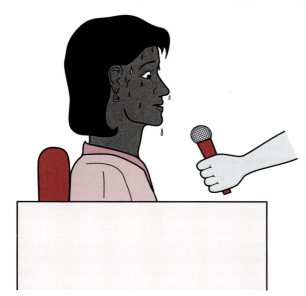

Fig. 2.3 Speaking in a key situation such as before a jury can also be a frightening experience, causing the body to respond as if a physical danger were present.

when speaking before a group is so intense that the body responds as if it were (Fig. 2.3). McQuade and Aikman also list two other types of acute stress that cause a primal body reaction.

The second primal stress is the basic problem of obtaining food. This type of threat does not elicit a fight-or-flight response but rather persuasion, bartering, searching, and producing. Although the stress resulting from a threat to the food supply is seldom life threatening to us today, it is a psychologic stress that may be as painful as hunger itself. You learned in infancy that while receiving food, you also received attention, which you translated as receiving love; you were receiving more than the basic nutrients for life. When food is withheld, you may feel that recognition, attention, and love are also being withheld.

Death, the third primal stress, is inevitable. For many people, a philosophic or religious belief provides an anchor in times of turmoil and stress. The unalterable truth is that someday you will die. In the meantime, you should make your life worth living and become the person you want to be.

Coping with life stresses is not new to you. While growing and developing, you made many adjustments and concessions. You learned to distinguish your father, mother, brother, and sister, and finally you realized that you were not any of them—this was your discovery of yourself. Later in childhood, you began exploring and discovered that you could control parts of your world. You learned what was

dangerous and what was safe, what belonged to you and what belonged to others, and that certain behavior brought rewards whereas other behavior was punished. While you were learning these things, you were developing patterns for coping with life situations. Your behavior was based on your most satisfying experiences. It may sound simplistic, but most people behave in a manner that will give them something in return that will satisfy their basic human needs.

B. F. Skinner, a twentieth century educational psychologist, studied animal and human behavior. He found that when placed in a **controlled environment** (i.e., an artificial environment to verify the results of an experiment), animals could be taught to perform complex acts by rewarding the desired behavior. He called this **reinforcement behavior**. He found that behavior could also be modified through punishment or merely with the absence of a reward. Skinner later worked with humans under less-controlled conditions. He found that a form of the reinforcement theory could be applied to shape and modify human behavior.

STRESS AND CONFLICT

Stress

Stress is a response that can occur when your behavior or that of another fails to produce the desired or expected results. Although you should expect a moderate amount of stress throughout life, a disproportionate amount of stress may occur during your first year away from home. A primary source of stress during adolescence and early adulthood occurs when the need to assert your independence does not produce the expected results in a world that requires a balance between independence and dependence. You must face the problem of needing to be both dependent and independent at the same time. The life situations that require a balance between dependence and independence are many. A financial base is necessary for independent living; however, even with wealth, a totally independent existence is impossible. You will always be dependent on others to a certain degree. Most employment opportunities are authoritarian in nature, which means that workers depend on supervisors, and supervisors depend on managers. Regardless of how independent you wish to be, you still have dependent needs; therefore you must accept those aspects of life that involve interdependence. You learn to submit to rational authority and at the same time retain a degree of independence.

Conflict

Conflict is the tension that results from disagreements between incompatible needs or drives, either within you or with others. Conflict does not have to be open warfare or an outbreak of hostilities. It can be as mild and benign as a difference of opinion or diversity in taste. Conflict is an inescapable part of living, and, generally speaking, the closer and more intimate the relationship, the greater the opportunities for conflict. Conflict can be either healthy and constructive or hostile and destructive. Conflicts occur in families, among close friends, in work relationships, in student groups, and even among strangers.

A type of conflict that is increasingly important concerns identity and role assignment. In the past, roles were often assigned by society; male and female roles were clearly defined. Today, people are questioning their assigned roles and are independently seeking their own identities. This is a source of conflict for both sexes for which there is no magic formula. It calls for understanding, tolerance, and patience.

Another category of conflict concerns your perceptions of encroachment on your territory. For example, nonsmokers may be offended by cigarette smoke, or a roommate may disturb you by playing the radio too loudly. Persuasion, tact, diplomacy, and compromise may be required in these situations.

Managing and Resolving Conflict

Some types of conflicts are more easily resolved than others. Factual issues are simpler to resolve than value or identification issues. The most important factor in resolving conflict is to attack the issue rather than the individual. You should focus on the issue and resist any temptation to criticize or demean the other person; remember, a true victory is one in which the relationship remains intact and both people are satisfied with the results.

Resolving conflict with casual acquaintances is different from resolving conflict with family and friends. With casual acquaintances, you are less concerned about maintaining goodwill. The fear of damaging the relationship is slight or perhaps nonexistent. With family and close friends, your desire to maintain the relationship is more intense. Consequently, emotions and feelings influence your behavior. Compromise, participation, and allowance for imperfections are elements that you will have to use in resolving conflicts with others and within yourself.

Internal conflict may be as damaging and destructive as the tense encounters you have with others. With others, you can use the inherent fight-or-flight response. Whether you choose fight or flight, your action is clearly defined and directed. Dealing with conflict within yourself is more difficult. You cannot run away from yourself, and to fight yourself is unproductive. To maintain a low-stress lifestyle, you must learn to control the factors that are at the root of tension and anxiety.

Silber and Glim (1981) list seven ways people behave when confronted with conflict: they attack, internalize, deny, isolate, manipulate, withdraw, or confront. These authors suggest confronting the problem in a mature manner in open dialogue. Feelings of empathy are created between two people when they share risks, dangers, doubts, and insecurities. Emotions must be dealt with to bring about a change in behavior. Negative emotions serve as a barrier and must be confronted to resolve the conflict. Silber and Glim also state that you must trust the other person when trying to resolve conflict and you must be open and honest about your objectives, expectations, and needs.

The first step in resolving any conflict is identifying the cause of the conflict. In some cases, the cause may be a simple difference of opinion. Factual issues can usually be resolved by accepting the opinion of an authority on the issue. Issues involving values, such as differences in religion, politics, or ethics, are more difficult; a clear-cut answer is unlikely. Facts related to values may be questioned or interpreted differently. For example, a religious writing may be considered to be the authority, but the interpretation of that writing may vary considerably.

Examine the way you have organized your life. Stress and tension can result from the failure to organize your life in a way that is comfortable for you. Pacing your work and study will prevent a sense of urgency and help you keep up with your obligations in a more relaxed manner.

Planning, setting objectives, listing activities for reaching objectives, and scheduling work and recreation should reduce stress. Regular use of a calendar, either print or electronic, is an invaluable tool in planning and staying organized. Making improvements in your performance through discipline and motivation should improve your chances of minimizing anxiety, tension, and conflict. The aim is to create a healthier, happier self and to find serenity, meaning, and wholeness in your life.

LEARNING HOW TO LEARN

As stated earlier in this chapter, learning how to learn is an important component in mastering the requirements of the radiography program. With the assumption that you have the ability to learn, this discussion is designed to help you use that ability more effectively.

Learning is a matter of storing information in memory and retrieving the information when needed. Storing information is not difficult. The sights and sounds of daily living are stored in memory with no particular effort. It is recall or retrieval from memory that is difficult. Educators have long known this; there was a time when **rote memorization**, which means learning word by word with little internalization, was a common practice in schools. This practice was due, in part, to the economic conditions of the time; only the youth had access to schools, and education ceased abruptly as the youth entered the labor market. Teachers believed they were educating for a lifetime; although the material might not be immediately understood because of the students' limited life experiences, they could rely on the memory-stored information to serve as the need arose.

Some educators thought that memorizing exercised the mind and thus increased the learning ability. The analogy was drawn from the effects of exercise on muscular tissue—an analogy that recent research suggests is valid.

Understanding does not occur without memory. The ability to think depends on information being stored in memory and on the ability to recover it and logically manipulate it. Curriculum design is based on the assumptions that students remember what has been learned and that advanced courses can build on knowledge stored in memory. So memorizing, even rote drilling, has again become respectable.

INTENTIONAL MEMORIZATION

Many things are stored in memory, some with conscious effort. Intentional memorization occurs in your deliberate pursuit of knowledge in a systematic or planned study situation. It can be divided into two parts: perception and attention.

Perception

If a scene is presented to a group of observers, each observer will probably perceive it in a different way. To make sense of it, each observer will try to match the scene with a similar scene or scenes stored in his or her memory. The observers are unaware that they are supplying data to make the scene fit into a similar scene or experience in their past. Thus how you perceive something is heavily influenced by what you have stored in memory. Memory also influences the accuracy of your **perceptions,** which are your observations and resultant mental images. In his experiments in the psychology of perception, Sir Frederick Bartlett found that line drawings that were even vaguely familiar to observers could be perceived and reproduced with greater accuracy than unfamiliar patterns. Thus the greater the amount of similar information stored in your memory, the more accurate your perceptions and recall of something new.

Suppose you have before you a familiar object, for example, a fish, and are asked to make a line drawing of it. You can probably produce a line drawing that is fairly recognizable to anyone (Fig. 2.4). You perceive the fish with its fins, scales, and gills. Now suppose marine biology students with a vast amount of knowledge about the particular species of fish undertake the same assignment. Their perceptions of

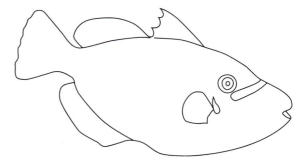

Fig. 2.4 Simple perceptual line drawing.

the object will no doubt be different. They will note the lateral fin spread, the positions of the upper and lower fins, the graduated arrangement of the scales, the medially deeply notched tail, and many other details that escape the eye of the untrained observer; their reproductions of their perceptions of the object will be more detailed and accurate (Fig. 2.5). This is an example of how things previously learned and stored in memory affect the perception of objects.

Attention

Attention means concentrating on one activity to the exclusion of others. One of the obvious ways to maintain attention is to eliminate interfering thoughts that come from distractions in the environment or from pressing problems. Many of the distractions in the environment can be controlled (e.g., loud noises, conversation or chatter, uncomfortable room temperature). Inner anxiety, fears, and persistent worry about personal and financial problems are distractions that are more difficult to eliminate. Realizing, however, that these distractions are probably the ones that are most seriously interfering with your ability to concentrate is important. A special effort should be made to discipline your mind. You may need to abandon your

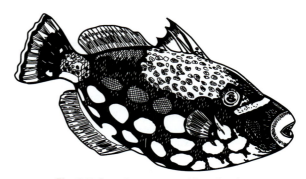

Fig. 2.5 Complex perceptual line drawing.

problem temporarily during learning sessions that require intense concentration. If the problem itself cannot be immediately solved, practice shelving it by refusing to give it conscious attention during periods that require intense concentration.

You can also improve your ability to concentrate by preparing to pay attention. Preparing involves creating a state of readiness; this means that you must prepare yourself to get the most from a class lecture, a laboratory demonstration, or a reading assignment. You may encounter lectures that seem dull, speakers who are boring, and reading material that is monotonous. You can add interest to a dull lecture by learning something about the subject and the speaker, if possible, before the lecture begins.

Working rapidly is another way to improve concentration. By this time, you probably have an idea of what your attention span is, so the objective is to maximize the effectiveness of your span. The adage, "what is rapidly learned is quickly forgotten; what is slowly learned is long remembered" has no basis. In fact, experiments have shown the reverse to be true. Rapid learning results in slow forgetting, and slow learning results in rapid forgetting. Working rapidly may require that you increase your listening and reading skills, as well as other mental activities.

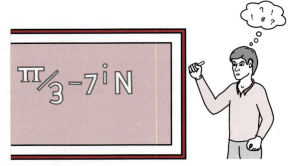

Fig. 2.6 Technical material that is new or appears too complicated requires forced concentration.

Improving Listening Skills

Educators have given a great deal of attention to improving reading skills. Only recently, however, has adequate attention been paid to the skill of listening. The research of Ralph Nichols and Ned Flanders of the University of Minnesota exemplifies this interest in listening skills; they report that people rarely listen with near-maximum efficiency. Nichols estimates that listeners operate at approximately a 25% level of efficiency when listening to a 10-minute talk. He found that Americans average 100 words per minute when speaking informally to an audience. The listener, however, listens at an easy cruising speed of 400 to 500 words per minute. Nichols concludes that the difference between speech speed and thought speed operates as a tremendous pitfall; it allows for increments of time in which the mind of the listener can wander.

Educators and psychologists have suggested some ways for improving listening skills:

1. Create an interest in what is being said. You must make an effort to find a motive or reason for listening so that you get in the right frame of mind.
2. Listen without prejudice and with an open mind (Fig. 2.6). You must guard against tuning out individuals whose ideas and beliefs are not congruent with your own. Your perceptions of the significance of the educator have an effect on how well you listen. Master teachers such as John Dewey and Maria Montessori are not encountered every day, but many educators are worth your listening efforts. Listening with an open mind is equally important with regard to subject matter. In this area, too, students tend to be selective. Details that do not fit comfortably with their notions and values are screened out.
3. Make written notes. Because you cannot remember every part of a lecture and you may unwittingly tune out certain uncomfortable parts, taking notes is important.

Improving Reading Skills

Improving reading skills requires far more than mere speed-reading techniques. *An efficient reader thinks, anticipates, and evaluates while reading.* Reading is a complex intellectual process with no magic formula. Some basic principles, however, can be used to increase your reading speed without sacrificing comprehension:

1. Quickly scan through the reading material to familiarize yourself with the organization and structure of the body of thought.
2. Develop a clear idea of what you expect to learn. Ask yourself what information you expect to learn and what questions are likely to be answered.
3. Search for the main ideas. Generally, the first sentence of a paragraph gives the main thought; the sentences that follow are a further development of the idea.

Practice exercises may increase your concentration while reading. When reading technical and scientific materials, the exercise that will probably be the most helpful is the practice of recall. Recall is a simple exercise performed by reading a page and then, with the page covered, trying to recall as much of the material as possible. Recall what you have read by reciting it aloud. Reciting gives you the benefit of both hearing and voicing the material, and involving the senses enhances the memory. Reciting aloud is probably the best test of how well you understand the material. Continue to practice the technique until you feel confident in your progress. This exercise not only improves your reading skills, but it is also one of the best ways of increasing your memory power.

RETRIEVING FROM MEMORY

Psychologists make a distinction between short-term memory and long-term memory. Remembering a telephone number just long enough to dial it is an example of short-term memory. It is transient and fleeting, and it fades rapidly. Long-term memory is more permanent memory storage (i.e., the recording of memory facts, images, sounds, pleasure, pain, and other life experiences), and it is the subject of this discussion about memory retrieval, which is the recalling, recovering, or obtaining of events and experiences stored in memory.

Long-term memory seems to require more activity in the storing process that relates to the organization and association of the information. The organizing process is not fully understood, but an analogy may help. Think of your mind as a file into which you place all previously acquired data under the appropriate subject headings. The filing of information continues with each new item placed with the associated data previously stored. In time, some of the files contain large quantities of information, and they expand and bulge with the sheer volume of items; other files may receive only a few items of information, and others may receive none. The files that increase only slightly or that do not increase at all may be displaced to make room for the more voluminous ones. Indeed, an inactive file may become lost or may at least require considerable effort to locate. Storage and retrieval in memory may be similar. This is a simple analogy to apply to something as complex as the human memory, but it should serve to make a point: the more facts you associate with an item of information, the more permanent the storage of the item in memory, and the more accessible that item becomes.

Donald and Eleanor Laird, in their *Techniques for Efficient Remembering*, offer some helpful suggestions for retrieving facts from memory. *Having a mental set for remembering* is their first suggestion, which means that you intend to remember and resolve to remember information that you know will be useful.

Reacting actively is their second suggestion; that is, talk and think about the information; make an application, if possible; and rehearse, recite, and interpret what you have learned.

Refreshing your memory is the third suggestion. Forgetting occurs rather rapidly despite our best efforts to remember. Refreshing or touching up a fading memory reinforces the learning process, which is particularly important with unfamiliar technical material.

Searching for meaning is the fourth—and probably most important—suggestion. Searching for meaning will increase your concentration and thus aid in memorization.

FORGETTING

Understanding why you forget will help you to understand how you remember. Forgetting is frustrating when you are trying to pass a test, recall the name of an acquaintance, or solve a pressing problem. You must realize, however, that forgetting is essential to survival. Suppose you could not forget. Imagine what life would be like if all the pains of a lifetime remained fresh in your memory. Think of the mental and emotional anguish you have experienced and add to this the physical pain of illness and trauma. Suppose none of this faded and the sharp reality of every painful experience was as vivid in your memory now as when it occurred. Nature has marvelous ways of protecting you, and forgetting is one method. This survival mechanism allows you to partially—but not entirely—forget pain.

The inability to forget painful experiences entirely has its positive aspects. It is essential to survival. Remembering the painful consequence of touching a hot stove, jumping from an extreme height, or being hit by a moving or flying object gives direction to your action and allows you to order the safety of your environment.

Forgetting: Pain, Pleasure

The scale from pain to pleasure is a broad one. In the middle of the extremes lies a neutral ground that cannot be identified as painful or pleasant. Some experiences that are neither painful nor particularly pleasant may be interpreted as merely insignificant; this may account for the common failure to remember names, dates, places, and material you do not understand. You seldom forget the name of a significant person or the date and place of a happily anticipated event. When the pleasure-anticipation level is high, you are able to remember with no difficulty. You can even recall pleasurable experiences that happened years ago. Conversely, you tend to forget events associated with embarrassment, disappointment, or other unpleasant feelings. In effect, you can will yourself to forget unpleasant experiences and to remember the pleasant ones.

If it is true that you forget, by design, unpleasant things and remember pleasant things, then why do you sometimes forget what you want to remember? What you want to remember is perceived as pleasant in that it will help you pass an examination, solve a problem, or make a decision. So why does it take so much effort? Forgetting and remembering are activities far too complex to fit neatly into a pain–pleasure concept. However, taking a commonsense approach should help you identify and analyze your own pattern of remembering. This does not mean that you have to enjoy all the material you must commit to memory to remember it.

Errors in Remembering

Human beings have a way of altering and distorting the details of a remembered event. You seldom remember factual details of an event, a speech, or reading material. Some things are incorrectly remembered, for example, where the car is parked. You correctly remember that the car is parked in the parking garage, but you incorrectly think that it is parked on the third level, when in fact it is on the fourth level. You have noticed how the size of the fish caught by the hopeful fisherman increases with each telling or how the brawl in the beer parlor increases in drama at each recounting. Perhaps the most common example of distortion of memory is in reminiscing about the "good old days." It is not generally remembered that the "good old days" did not include refrigeration, washing machines, television, reliable automobiles, penicillin, polio vaccine, and other things that today's technology makes possible. Memory does not fade uniformly. Some parts of memory remain to hold together the general structure, but the details are often missing or altered.

Some motive for twisting and distorting the reality of events and experiences must exist. Indeed, two well-confirmed explanations for errors in memory are offered. One is that you distort and retouch memories to make the details more in keeping with what you wish were so; this distortion helps you support your beliefs, values, notions, and hopes and defends your prejudices. The second explanation is that you add detail to your recollection of an event in a way that seems reasonable to you to complete and make sense of a sketchy or incomplete recollection; it is simply more satisfying to fill in and round out the missing details to achieve wholeness.

Inaccurate remembering cannot be eliminated altogether, but cutting it down to some extent is possible. The most obvious safeguard against inaccurate recall is to memorize well. Taking notes is essential for safeguarding important facts and information that must be recalled precisely. Understanding your prejudices and biases, as well as your hopes, dreams, and aspirations, can guard against wishful remembering. The most important safeguard is to understand clearly from the start so that fallacies in thinking will not occur.

The following is a list of recommended practices that will help you optimize your memory's performance:

1. Give the cerebral cells an opportunity to rest and rejuvenate, which can be done by getting a sufficient amount of sleep and relaxation.
2. Provide the brain with sufficient nutrients to meet the requirements of the cells. Proper nutrition cannot be overemphasized. Research indicates that the brain tires less easily when it receives glucose derived from protein rather than from carbohydrates.
3. Schedule your study periods at a time when you are most alert and attentive.
4. Organize your environment so that distractions are reduced and attention can be focused on the material to be learned.
5. Read for meaning, and intend to memorize.

Understanding Critical Thinking

All health care providers must be able to make logical decisions and wise choices; it goes without saying. The care of the patient demands that good judgment is exercised in the selection of technical factors for quality imaging and in other patient care tasks. You will be responsible for giving the physician a radiograph that is diagnostically sound and for providing safe care to the patient while performing the examination.

NEED FOR CRITICAL THINKING

As a professional, you will be making vital decisions regarding your own career. You will need to make choices regarding the route you follow in the profession to meet your own personal needs and goals.

What Is Critical Thinking?

Many definitions have been given for **critical thinking**. One definition calls it emancipatory learning. **Emancipation** means freedom from restraint or influence. Things that restrain or influence people can be personal, institutional, or environmental. Personal beliefs, rules and regulations of institutions, and physical environments can all work to prevent people from seeing new directions and gaining understanding and control of their own lives and of the world around them. **Emancipatory learning** means that learners become aware of the forces that have created the circumstances of their lives and take action to change them.

Another definition for critical thinking focuses on the use of morality and virtues, making wise judgments about aspects of our lives, and recognizing the impact these judgments will have on others. Some stress the importance of recognizing reality in the context of cultural elements and the process of trying to create order in a changing world.

Creating order in a changing world will be a challenge for us all. Never in our history have changes occurred with such rapidity. Global information and communication exchange, worldwide exchange of goods and services, and, most important, an exchange of ideas affect our world. Geographic boundaries are becoming blurred, as are the cultures and traditions of separate groups. Learning how to live and work in this changing world makes critical thinking more important than ever.

Although the wording of the definitions of critical thinking may differ, they are all made on the assumption that a set of values exists. Each definition assumes that these values are universal; for example, life is better than death, wellness is better than illness, happiness is better than sadness, pleasure is better than pain, and hope is better than despair. Therefore when we speak of making wise judgments, we have to agree on a set of values. These values are not unique to a specific culture or religion nor are they characteristic of a specific nation or state. They are universal except in rare aberrations of individuals, cult groups, and other deviants.

The assumption that you have accepted these values is a fair conclusion because you have chosen to be a health care provider. We may disagree on the specifics of behaviors that will best accomplish the preservation of these values, but if we disagree on the values, then further discussion is no longer needed. When we speak of making wise decisions, we are judging decisions made within the framework of a value system that is universally understood. It is equated with logical reasoning abilities and reflective judgment.

Qualities of a Critical Thinker

Critical thinkers are valued for their ability to look at a situation from a variety of perspectives. They are able to discern the best possible way to react to a situation, making them ideally suited for work in the health care profession. Box 2.1 summarizes the characteristics that a critical thinker needs to possess.

One of the first traits that one observes in critical thinkers is the presence of heart as well as mind. The definitions regarding critical thinking are reflective of human values and can thus be expected of critical thinkers. Such a thinker will be able to balance compassion with realism.

The critical thinker must also be analytical, which means finding evidence in unclear and confusing situations. Being alert to the consequences of accepting a course of action and being able to defend that position are both important.

Rushing into a plan without examining the ramifications of hastened actions can be dangerous.

Rational thinkers recognize reality; they can discern what is factual and true from what is opinion or misinformation. Seeking truth and making every effort to be honest with yourself is an important characteristic. To accomplish this, we must recognize the difference between what is true and what we wish were true. Making this distinction is more difficult than it may appear on the surface. Recognizing the laws of physics or mathematics as factual is simple enough; however, when the discussions involve government, religion, evolution, or other similar topics, facts become blurred and clouded with emotion. The truth is often elusive, and the evidence is less convincing. Nonetheless, critical thinkers seek to make rational judgments and act responsibly.

Open-mindedness is an important quality and necessary in the field of patient care. Disagreements are common, but a heated confrontation can be diffused by the willingness of the critical thinker to listen and understand, which is especially important in dealing with patients. Attempting to understand a patient's point of view will leave him or her feeling more secure that his or her health care provider actually cares. Dealing with diversity while remaining true to your values is often complicated, but patience and compromise can lead to a solution.

Patience and organization allow time for the critical thinker to gather evidence, test ideas, and systematically work through tough problems and complex questions. Rash judgments are less likely to be made when time is taken to internalize or ponder the question. During this time, ideas can be tested to ensure that a logical and just decision can be made or an appropriate action can be taken. The critical thinker resists the desire to reach a solution before all the facts are in.

An inquisitive nature leads a critical thinker to seek knowledge from many sources. This quality is found in all effective learners. The need to learn, to gather information, and to use that information wisely is a sign of growth and maturity.

In light of these qualities of a critical thinker, it becomes obvious that becoming a critical thinker is a process. Unlike a characteristic you are born with, critical thinking is developed throughout life by the experiences you encounter.

FACTORS THAT HINDER CRITICAL THINKING

Background Beliefs

Religious training, attitudes of society, cultural traditions, and teachings of our parents and school teachers form our background beliefs. These beliefs are the stabilizing forces that guide us and the glue that holds our society together. Often, they are the most deeply ingrained beliefs and thus the most intensely defended. Times occur,

BOX 2.1	**Characteristics of a Critical Thinker**
Human	
Analytical	
Rational	
Open-minded	
Systematic	
Inquisitive	

however, when these beliefs may be challenged by a conflicting value. If a physician must choose between performing an abortion to save a mother's life and defending his religious convictions that forbid it, to which does his obligation belong? Although no clear-cut answer to this question or others like it can usually be found, examining one's views and beliefs while keeping in mind the reality of the situation enables the critical thinker to choose the best solution.

Faulty Reasoning

Faulty reasoning occurs when biased or false information is stated as fact. Often, this is the aim of advertising. Frequently, celebrities and famous athletes are used as spokespeople for a certain product or service. The logic here is that an endorsement by a public figure will lend credibility to the advertiser's claims that the product is the best. In this case, the ultimate goal is persuading you to buy the product.

If your only evidence of the worth of the information is because of an "authority" endorsement, it is time to examine the information more critically. Even statistics can be used to persuade. We reason that statistics are accurate and unquestionable. However, the interpretation of the statistics may be faulty. Statistics must be examined from several aspects such as sample size, evidence of bias, nature of the information, and even how recently the information was gathered. Some statistics, such as those regarding spousal abuse or rape, are by their very nature hard to obtain because most incidences go unreported. Statistics are also used to predict the future, with the assumption that what happened in the past will be repeated in the future. This assumption may or may not be true. Although some statistics may be suspect, we should not dismiss using them altogether, but it does mean we must critically examine them and understand their limitations.

Group Loyalty

The natural cohesiveness in a social group is called the **herd instinct**. In such groups, a desire to gain status within the group exists. Generally, all members follow a predetermined set of acceptable behaviors. Success in everyday life depends to a great extent on being accepted by your social group, a concept that is learned early in life. This instinct keeps us loyal to the group; consequently, we tend to behave in ways that will enhance our status and make us feel comfortable within the group. At a more primitive level, instinct makes us aware that our survival depends on the survival of the group. Believing what others in the group believe and defending these beliefs without examining or testing them are natural.

For the most part, loyalty is beneficial to the preservation of the group, but when horrifying acts are committed by mobs or street gangs, loyalty becomes disastrous. In recognizing the natural tendency to group loyalty, we must also realize that this loyalty tends to make us see everything in terms of our own social group. This view may hinder our ability to make just and logical decisions. Unfortunately, creative ideas can be stifled in a group environment.

Frozen Mind-Set

Individuals with frozen minds reach frozen solutions. This argument is centered in maintaining the status quo. They find the status quo comfortable because they think, often times rightly so, that they have the consensus and support of the group. Early in childhood, we learn to go along with the group and base our actions on group approval. Maintaining the status quo is so deeply ingrained in some people that no amount of evidence will change their minds. It takes courage to recognize this mind-set within ourselves, and it takes discipline to weigh the evidence and create a better solution.

Emotional Baggage

Almost all of us have issues they feel strongly about and will defend vigorously. Emotions run high in the discussions of these issues, and sometimes logic is abandoned. The key to keeping your emotions in check is to identify the issues that cause you discomfort or ire when discussions run counter to your opinion. Some issues to which many have emotional ties are abortion, gun control, the death penalty, censorship—the list goes on and on.

When you have identified the issue that causes you to feel anger or discomfort, it helps to seek out information on both sides of the argument. Learn why those whose position runs counter to yours believe the way they do and on what basis their opinions rest. Make an effort to talk to people whose opinions differ from your own and read articles on the subject in newspapers, magazines, and books. Understanding both sides of an issue will help sharpen your skills in critical thinking. Developing a greater understanding in no way means that you should change your opinions to conform to the views of others, but it does mean that you can more calmly weigh the evidence so that logic, rather than emotion, determines your actions.

BECOMING A CRITICAL THINKER
Humility

The first step in becoming a critical thinker is to take a humble approach and be open to learning. It is acceptable, even admirable, to admit that you are not sure or that you need more information. You are living at a time when people are pressured to give quick answers; to examine or consider other points of view is often criticized. Short, quick answers are easy to come by when speaking of things that are certain, such as a mathematical answer. For example, you do not need to seek other points of view to determine that the square root of 144 is 12. Such a factual answer leaves no element of doubt. Answers to other questions are more difficult because of uncertainty or the presence of doubt. In cases in which a consensus is widely held in your group, giving up your belief and accepting another view can be difficult. Take, for example, the commonly held belief that more money spent on education will result in higher test scores and therefore a better education. Reflecting on this statement reveals two beliefs that need to be further examined. First, we should question whether money alone is the answer or whether how it is used makes the difference. Second, we should examine the belief that higher scores mean better education. Could higher scores merely be the result of lowering the level of difficulty of the examinations? These two examples, one of certainty, and the other of widely held beliefs, make it necessary to distinguish truths and certainties from beliefs and opinions.

Respect for Others

Another stage in becoming a critical thinker is learning to respect the opinions of others. To live peacefully in a diverse society, we must be tolerant of many different cultures and traditions. Just as geographic lines have been blurring, cultural and traditional lines have also been blurring. At times, this creates a dilemma because tradition is mingled with religion and is a part of every civilized society. Logic and wisdom will, at this point, be needed.

Self-Awareness

Recognize the things that make you glad, the things that make you sad, and the things that make you mad. Although this is a simplistic way of examining your personality, it is a start. As you grow and develop in your critical thinking ability, the issues that bring forth an emotional response will become more evident, and you will be able to deal with them more effectively. When you are aware of your own standards and ethical values, you can make objective decisions and act responsibly.

Honing Your Skills

It takes practice to become proficient in activities such as sports, music, and dance. Practice will also help you develop your skills in critical thinking. As issues arise, consciously and deliberately examine them from several points of view and weigh the evidence on the most reliable and convincing basis. This will enable you to resist making instant judgments and taking rash actions.

CONCLUSION

Becoming a better student requires effort, but understanding yourself, your needs, your aspirations, and your perception of the world around you will enable you to order your activities in a practical and logical manner.

Mastering effective ways to better your skills in reading, listening, and storing and retrieving information in memory will ensure success in becoming a better student. These skills will allow you to proceed with confidence, not only in your radiography program but also throughout your career.

Characteristics of critical thinkers are compassion, patience, respect for others' opinions, open-mindedness, and the ability to be analytical. As a health care provider, you will be confronted with many issues requiring logical judgment and rational action. Critical thinkers are aware of their values and know the reason and consequences of the actions taken.

QUESTIONS FOR DISCUSSION AND CRITICAL THINKING

1. Discuss the importance of being aware of one's human needs.
2. Given the complexity of clinical education, explain why managing stress and conflict resolution are important to your success.
3. Describe the importance of understanding learning, listening, and reading to your success as a radiography student.
4. Explain the role of short-term and long-term memory in the learning process.
5. Discuss critical thinking and how it can be applied in the classroom and clinical settings.
6. Explain factors that hinder critical thinking and how they can be managed.

BIBLIOGRAPHY

Alessandra A, Hunsaker P. *Communicating at work.* New York: Simon & Schuster; 1993.

Bartlett F. *Remembering, a study in experimental and social psychology.* New York: Cambridge University Press; 1964.

Charles CM. *Educational psychology: the instructional endeavor.* ed 2. St. Louis: Mosby; 1976.

Cohen G, Kiss G, Voi LM. *Memory current issues.* ed 2. Philadelphia: Open University Press; 1993.

Coles GS. *The learning mystique, a critical look at learning disabilities.* New York: Pantheon Books; 1987.

Coles R. *The moral intelligence of children.* New York: Random House; 2001.

Coury V. *Personal communication* (compiled for course supplement). Memphis: University of Tennessee Center for the Health Sciences; 1982.

Diestler S. *Becoming a critical thinker: a user friendly manual.* ed 3. New York: Prentice Hall; 2011.

Ellis D. *Becoming a master student.* ed 16. Boston, MA: Wadsworth; 2017.

Fulghum R. *From beginning to end, the rituals of our lives.* New York: Villard Books; 1996.

Gordon S. *Psychology for you.* New York: Oxford; 1974.

James W. The principles of psychology. In: *The works of William James.* Cambridge, MA: Harvard University Press; 1981.

Kahne H, Cavender N. *Logic and contemporary rhetoric.* ed 13. Boston, MA: Wadsworth; 2017.

Laird DA, Laird EC. *Techniques for efficient remembering.* New York: McGraw-Hill; 1960.

Maslow AH. A theory of human motivation. *Psychol Rev.* 1943; 50:370.

McQuade W, Aikman A. *Stress—what it is—what it can do to your health—how to fight back.* New York: Bantam Books; 1975.

Morse R, Furst ML. *Stress for success: a holistic approach to stress and its management.* New York: Van Nostrand Reinhold; 1979.

Nichols RG. *Listening is good business,* vol 1, no 2, Ann Arbor, MI. In: *Bureau of Industrial Relations.* School of Business Administration: The University of Michigan; 1962.

Ormrod JE. *Human learning.* ed 7. New York: Pearson; 2015.

Silber M, Glim J. *We-ism world of the 80s. Pace Magazine*; 1981. May/June.

Skinner BF. *Science and human behavior.* New York: McMillan; 1960.

Small G. *The memory prescription: Dr. Gary Small's 14-day plan to keep your brain and body young.* New York: Hyperion; 2004.

Tye M. *The imagery debate.* Boston: Massachusetts Institute of Technology; 1991.

3

Evolution of Health Care Delivery

OBJECTIVES

On completion of this chapter, you should be able to:

- List the main contributions to medicine from ancient Egypt, India, China, and Greece.
- Describe the medical practice of the ancient Hebrews.
- Outline the teachings of Hippocrates.
- Describe the effect of Christianity on medicine.
- List events during the Renaissance that were significant in the progress of medicine.
- Describe important advances in medicine from the eighteenth and nineteenth centuries.
- List the significant developments in medicine during the twentieth century.
- Indicate trends in medicine for the twenty-first century.
- Describe the major issues in medicine at the present time.
- Define disease.
- List the top 10 causes of death in the United States.
- Compare mortality rates among various groups.
- List the primary disabling conditions present in US society.

- List diseases that have been eradicated or are targeted for elimination.
- Explain the significance of emerging infectious diseases.
- List key social forces that affect the health care system.
- Discuss the dominant ethical issues in medicine today.
- Explain the impact of an aging population on health care delivery.
- Describe the nation's health care expenditures.
- Explain prospective payment.
- Correlate defensive medicine, medical malpractice, and health care costs.
- Give the top five causes of death, and list the associated risk factors.
- Describe a typical wellness program.
- Describe the advantages of giving up smoking.
- Link poor diet to major causes of death.
- Outline dietary guidelines for good health.
- Discuss the role of the radiologic technologist in patient education.

OUTLINE

Prehistoric and Ancient Medicine
Ancient Egypt
Ancient India
Ancient China
Ancient Greece
 Pre-Hippocratic Medicine
 Hippocrates
Christianity
The Renaissance
Eighteenth Century
Nineteenth Century
Twentieth Century
Twenty-first Century

Health and Disease
 Life Expectancy
 Mortality
 Morbidity
 Emerging Infectious Diseases
Social Forces That Affect Health Care
Ethical Issues
Economic Forces That Affect Health Care
 Health Spending by Major Sources of Funds
Need for Health Care Management
Preventive Medicine
Health Care System
Beginning of Your Challenge
Conclusion

KEY TERMS

defensive medicine	epidemic	mortality
diet	health	pandemic
disease	health maintenance organizations	prospective payment system
emerging infectious diseases	morbidity	smoking

PREHISTORIC AND ANCIENT MEDICINE

The history of medicine abounds with tales of cooperation and confrontation with nature. Disease was present on earth long before human life, and we can only speculate about the human practice of prehistoric medicine. Fractures were probably common injuries. Egyptian mummies and radiographic images of the *ice man* show characteristics of arteriosclerosis, pneumonia, urinary infections, stones, parasites, cavities, teeth erosion, abscesses, pyorrhea, arthritis, and tubercular disease of the spine. Prehistoric people probably treated their wounds similarly to the way animals treat themselves: immersing themselves in cool water and applying mud to irritated areas, sucking stings, licking wounds, and exerting pressure on wounds to stop the bleeding.

Until well into the nineteenth century, medical treatment was intertwined with religion and magic (Fig. 3.1). Some cultures treated their sick, elderly, and disabled with kindness. Other cultures, during times of famine, sent the elders out into the unsheltered environment; some even killed and ate disabled tribe members. Disease was thought to be caused by gods and spirits, and magic was used to drive away evil forces. Tribal healers held high political and social positions and were responsible for performing religious ceremonies and protecting the tribe from bad weather, poor harvests, and catastrophes. Along with sucking, cupping, bleeding, fumigating, and steam baths, medicinal herbs were used to treat wounds. Surgery

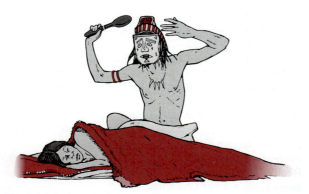

Fig. 3.1 Magic and religion played an important role in medicine well into the nineteenth century.

was used to treat bone fractures and to sew up wounds. The Mesopotamians studied hepatoscopy, which is the detailed examination of the liver. They believed the liver was the seat of life and the collecting point of blood. Although gods and magic still played an important role in medicine, rational thought about nature's relationship to health began to increase.

The ancient Hebrews still considered disease to be divine punishment and a mark of sin. Plagues and epidemics such as leprosy were often mentioned in the Bible, as were medications such as balsams, gums, spices, oils, and narcotics. Surgery was performed only under ritual circumstances.

Hebrew medicine was influenced by the Greeks around the fourth century BC with an emphasis placed on anatomy and physiology, diet, massage, and drugs. Disease was considered an imbalance of the four humors of the body: phlegm, blood, yellow bile, and black bile.

ANCIENT EGYPT

The deities of ancient Egypt were associated with health, illness, and death. Isis was the healing goddess, Hathor was the mistress of heaven and the protector of women during childbirth, and Keket ensured fertility.

The embalming practices of the Egyptians have provided much of our knowledge of ancient medicine. The most elaborate embalming practice required that the liver, lungs, stomach, and intestines be preserved in stone jars so that they could function for eternity. Cranial contents were removed with hooks through the nostrils. The skull and abdominal cavities were washed with spices; soaked for 70 days in a solution of clay and salts of carbonate, sulfate, and chloride; and then washed. The corpse was then coated with gums and wrapped in fine linen.

The ancient Egyptians linked anatomy and physiology with theology—each body part had a special deity as its protector. They believed that the body was composed of a system of channels, with the heart at the center. They thought air came in through the ears and nose, entered the channels, went to the heart, and was then delivered to the rest of the body. They believed the channels also carried blood, urine, feces, tears, and sperm.

Although the main water source, the Nile River, was probably clean in ancient Egypt, public health was also a concern. Egyptian homes were immaculate, and personal hygiene was practiced regularly. The prevalent diseases included intestinal ailments, malaria, trachoma, night blindness, cataracts, arteriosclerosis, and epidemic diseases. Diagnoses were made by probing wounds with fingers; taking the pulse; and studying sputum, urine, and feces. Religious rituals were still part of the healing process, as were drugs administered in the forms of pills, cake suppositories, enemas, ointments, drops, gargles, fumigations, and baths. Drugs were made from vegetable, mineral, and animal substances and imported materials such as saffron, cinnamon, perfumes, spices, sandalwood, gums, and antimony.

ANCIENT INDIA

The ancient Indians believed (as do many contemporary Indians) that life is an eternal cycle of creation, preservation, and destruction. Their religion allowed secular medicine and sound, rational health care practices, which is remarkable in light of their emphasis on the spiritual over the material. They detected diabetes by the sweetness of the patient's urine and treated snakebites by applying tourniquets. Surgery was a common procedure on the nose, earlobes, harelips, and hernias; it was also used to remove bladder stones and to perform amputations. The Indians also performed cesarean sections.

ANCIENT CHINA

In ancient China, harmony was considered to be a delicate balance between *yin* and *yang*, and Tao was considered *the way*. Illness was seen as a result of disregard for Tao or acting contrary to natural laws. Chinese medicine focused on the prevention of disease (Fig. 3.2). Because Confucius forbade any violation of the body, dissections were not performed in China until the eighteenth century. According to Nei Ching, five methods of treatment were available: cure the spirit; nourish the body; give medications; treat the whole body; and use acupuncture and moxibustion, which is a treatment similar to acupuncture in which a powdered plant is burned on the skin. Treatment came in the forms of exercise, physical therapy, massage, and administering medicinal herbs, trees, insects, stones, and grains. By the eleventh century, the Chinese had developed an inoculation against smallpox.

ANCIENT GREECE

In the sixth century BC, the Greeks built the healing temples of Asclepios in Thessaly. The temples contained a statue of

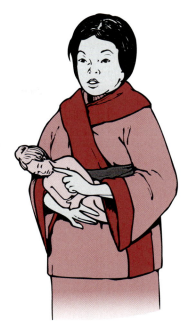

Fig. 3.2 For reasons of modesty, women in ancient China used figurines to indicate the location of their symptoms.

a god to whom gifts were often given as a sign of worship. Usually, a round building, the tholos, encircled a pool or sacred spring of water for purification. The abaton was a building considered to be an incubation site, where the cure took place. The patient went to sleep there until visited and cured by the god. The temples usually consisted of a theater, a stadium, a gymnasium, inns, and temporary housing. Healing rituals began after sundown and often involved fasting or abstinence from certain foods or wine.

Pre-Hippocratic Medicine

The ancient Greeks began applying scientific thought to medical theory very early. Thales (625–547 BC) professed that the basic element in all animal and plant life was water, from which came the earth and air. Anaximander (610–547 BC) believed that all living creatures originated in water. Anaximenes, born in 546 BC, believed that air was the element necessary for life. Heraclitus (540–480 BC) believed that fire was the principal element of life. By the sixth century BC, earth, air, fire, and water were accepted as the basic components of life on earth.

Hippocrates

During the sixth, fifth, and fourth centuries BC, the Greeks advanced medicine with their understanding of the place of humanity within the cosmos. Pythagoras, Empedocles, and

Democritus approached harmony with the universe in an objective, scientific manner. Mathematics, atomic theory, and the basic elements of nature were used to describe health and disease.

During this period, Hippocrates established himself as the *father of medicine*. His approach revolutionized medicine from the ancient past and began turning it into an objective science. Born around 460 BC, Hippocrates believed that people practicing medicine should be pure and holy. He taught that one should (1) observe all, (2) study the patient rather than the disease, (3) evaluate honestly, and (4) assist nature.

> *He employed few drugs and relied largely upon the healing powers of nature…. The treatment of disease for him was to assist and, above all, not to hinder nature. If succeeding generations had followed his precepts, patients would have been spared countless unnecessary operations and an enormous number of nauseous, disgusting, ineffectual and frequently harmful medicines (Major, 1954).*

Hippocrates' writings addressed mental illness, anxiety, and depression. His teachings reached a peak in Alexandria and then eventually penetrated the Roman Empire.

CHRISTIANITY

The dawn of Christianity changed many attitudes about medicine. Christians sought to bring the *healing message of Christ* to those in need. The Church dominated medicine during the Dark Ages, and practices involved prayer, exorcism, holy oil, relics of saints, supernaturalism, and superstition. At the same time, medical schools separate from the Church were established and soon became part of major universities.

During Jesus' personal ministry and that of his immediate followers, *healing* was not differentiated into physical, mental, or spiritual categories. The author of one of the Gospels was known as *Luke the physician*. The content of the Christian faith, with its emphasis on compassion, forgiveness, and concern for the unfortunate and the dispossessed, led the followers of Christianity to provide facilities for the care of the orphaned, elderly, outcast, and poor.

The Roman Emperor, Constantine, founded a hospital in the fourth century. Others were established by Christian communities in Caesarea, Edessa, and Bethlehem during the same century.

With the Crusades came the distribution of disease. In the twelfth century AD, Europe was inundated with leprosy, typhus, and smallpox. In 1347, bubonic plague spread through Europe and claimed nearly one fourth of its population.

THE RENAISSANCE

The Renaissance brought new beginnings in medicine. Paracelsus, the *father of pharmacology*, combined alchemy with the treatment of disease to produce a new science. Jean Fernel professed that physiology, pathology, and therapeutics were the standard disciplines of medicine; he was also the first to suggest that gonorrhea and syphilis were two separate diseases. Ambroise Paré was a forerunner in clinical surgery. An explosion of knowledge of human anatomy was led by Andreas Versalius; his dissections and drawings prompted his designation as the *father of anatomy*.

The seventeenth century was an age of scientific revolution. Latrochemistry, a combination of alchemy, medicine, and chemistry, was practiced by the followers of Paracelsus. Jan Baptista van Helmont made the first measurement of the relative weight of urine by comparing its weight with that of water. Galileo presented the laws of motion in a mathematical manner that could be applied to life on earth; Isaac Newton discovered gravity. William Harvey found that a continuous circulation of blood was present in a contained body system. Christian Huygens developed the centigrade system of measuring temperature; Gabriel Daniel Fahrenheit developed the system named after him for measuring temperature. Marcello Malpighi and Anton van Leeuwenhoek were forerunners in the invention of the microscope (Fig. 3.3). Quinine was discovered as a treatment for malaria. Leonardo da Vinci explored human anatomy through dissection; his anatomic sketches disseminated his findings.

EIGHTEENTH CENTURY

Significant discoveries continued into the eighteenth century. Albrecht von Haller did in-depth studies of the nervous system, discovered the relationship of the brain cortex to peripheral nerves, and became the founder of modern physiologic theory. Lazzaro Spallanzani discarded the theory of spontaneous generation and became a pioneer in experimental fertilization. Stephen Hales demonstrated the dynamics of blood circulation, stressed the importance of the capillary system, and became the first person to record blood pressure with a manometer.

The *father of pathology*, Giovanni Battista Morgagni, correlated anatomy with pathology. His research and writings laid the foundation for much of modern pathology.

Edward Jenner formulated the smallpox vaccination, which was considered one of the greatest discoveries in medical history. William Hunter, a specialist in obstetrics, founded the Great Windmill Street School of Anatomy, the first medical school in London. His brother, John Hunter, was a giant of the eighteenth century. An experimental surgeon, John Hunter developed a method of closing off

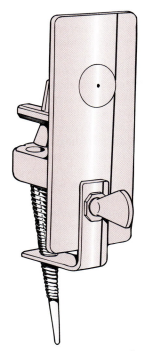

Fig. 3.3 Illustration of Leeuwenhoek's first microscope.

aneurysms, thus eliminating many unnecessary amputations. Hunter turned surgery into a respected science and became a pioneer in comparative anatomy.

The eighteenth century also saw dramatic changes in the care and treatment of mentally ill patients, with Phillippe Pinel demanding that a more humane regimen be instilled at Asylum de Bicêtre near Paris.

NINETEENTH CENTURY

Autopsies were the major focus of medicine during the nineteenth century. Carl Rokitansky was the most outstanding morphologic pathologist of his time. Rudolf Virchow professed that "all cells come from other cells" and revolutionized the understanding of cells. Claude Bernard was the founder of experimental physiology and discovered the principle of homeostasis, clarified the multiple functions of the liver, studied the digestive activities of the pancreas, and was the first to link the pancreas with diabetes. He pioneered and established the specialty of internal medicine.

René-Théophile Hyacinthe Laennec contributed to the pathologic and clinical understanding of chest diseases, including emphysema, bronchiectasis, and tuberculosis. He was also a pioneer in the invention and use of the stethoscope.

Surgery advanced in Paris during the French Revolution and Napoleonic wars. Ephraim McDowell performed the first successful abdominal operation to remove a huge cyst from an ovary. J. Marion Sims laid the foundation for gynecology and founded the Women's Hospital of the State of New York, the first institution of its kind. He also invented the Sims position and later the speculum and catheter.

By 1831, ether, nitrous oxide gas, and chloroform had been discovered but not yet applied to medical practice. After Joseph Priestley had discovered nitrous oxide gas, Humphry Davy suggested that it be used in surgery, but he was ignored. Although Crawford W. Long used sulfuric ether during surgery in 1842, he did not publicize its use. When anesthesia finally entered the world of surgery, surgical procedures multiplied in number and complexity. Joseph Lister discovered that bacteria were often the origin of disease and infection; thus safe surgical procedures were introduced to minimize the risks of surgery. Louis Pasteur discovered that the decay of food could be forestalled by heating the food and destroying harmful bacteria; he formulated the germ theory of disease and explained the effectiveness of asepsis and antisepsis.

Robert Koch performed extensive research into microorganisms and founded bacteriology. Psychiatry gained considerable respect from the work of Benjamin Rush, the first American psychiatrist. Based on his involved clinical studies of the human gastrointestinal tract, William Beaumont became the first prominent American physiologist. The foundation of modern genetics was laid by Gregor Mendel in 1886 with his experiments involving the heredity of plants.

November 8, 1895, is a date that forever changed the course of diagnoses of disease and injury. As will be explained more fully in Chapter 4, Wilhelm Roentgen discovered and described x-rays. Within months, the significance of these *new kinds of rays* in medicine was realized. Pierre and Marie Curie discovered radium 3 years later and provided the foundation for the use of radioactivity in the treatment of diseases.

Incredible as the discoveries of the previous centuries were, the twentieth century took medicine far beyond the dreams of the heartiest optimists of the past.

TWENTIETH CENTURY

Remarkable developments continued as the century turned and were built upon previous achievements. Major Walter Reed led a US Army board in discovering the cause of yellow fever, and this led to its eradication. Paul Ehrlich became the *father of chemotherapy*, which would have ramifications throughout the century. Pavlov conducted extensive research not only about the conditioned response but also about the process of digestion.

In 1913, Abel, Rowntree, and Turner invented the first artificial kidney, and this led to kidney dialysis. World War I provided the opportunity to explore wound infection in detail and advanced the prevention of surgical infections. Willem Einthoven made the first electrocardiogram, and Hans Burger used similar technology to invent the electroencephalogram. Lind, Eijkman, Hopkins, Szent-Gyorgyi, and Funk defined and isolated vitamins and described their role in the life process. This development would have a profound effect on diet and, late in the century, on the possible prevention and treatment of chronic diseases.

Surgical techniques were refined, and diagnostic procedures became more accurate. The invention of the electron microscope in 1930 (Fig. 3.4) made possible the study of viruses and advances in the fields of biochemistry, biophysics, physical chemistry, and immunology.

The Salk vaccine virtually eliminated the scourge of poliomyelitis (polio). Watson and Crick won a Nobel Prize in 1962 for accurately describing the deoxyribonucleic acid (DNA) molecule as a double helix and identifying its components. In 1967, Christiaan Barnard performed the first successful human heart transplant. In the ensuing years, other organs were successfully transplanted, adding another valuable tool to improving and saving lives.

Microminiaturization, which was invented for space travel, soon found its way into medicine. Coupled with evolving computer technology, the final 4 decades of the century vastly extended our abilities to diagnose and treat an entire array of medical conditions. Such electronics are used to monitor heart and brain activity with extreme accuracy. The marriage of computers and imaging equipment has provided digital radiography, computed tomography, and magnetic resonance imaging, and it has enhanced nuclear medicine and medical sonography. Treatment planning for radiation therapy is incredibly precise because of the use of computers.

Major organ transplants involving the heart, liver, lungs, and kidneys are performed today. Coronary bypass surgery is commonplace. Arthroscopic surgery works in the joint spaces of the body without major incisions. Laparoscopic surgery became commonplace for incisions into the abdomen for conditions affecting the gallbladder, kidneys, adrenal glands, and female reproductive system. Lithotripsy allows the painless passing of stones from the urinary system by first blasting them with sonic waves. Lasers are used routinely in countless procedures as a clean, painless way of removing growths; their accuracy allows their use in areas of the body where precision is indispensable.

Artificial hips and knees are inserted to replace those that are degenerating as a result of age or arthritis or that have been destroyed by injury. Plastic surgery allows the reconstruction of most areas of the body that have been disfigured as a result of disease or injury; it is also used extensively for elective cosmetic procedures.

TWENTY-FIRST CENTURY

The second millennium AD continues with a rapid expansion of technology and information. The accumulation of knowledge accelerates at an unprecedented pace, doubling every 15 to 18 months. Balancing this technologic explosion in medicine, a trend has emerged toward a more personal aspect of health care. The need for the human touch, caring, and concern has never been more important. More personal aspects of care such as the hospice movement for terminally ill patients and the reemergence of family practice as a specialty are but a couple of examples (Fig. 3.5). As you begin your studies in this intriguing profession, keep in mind that the human aspect of patient care and quality service must be ever present in your practice.

Research into genetics has greatly expanded our knowledge about heredity. The entire DNA code has now been deciphered, and this has opened a new era in the treatment and prevention of disease. The unfortunate affliction of

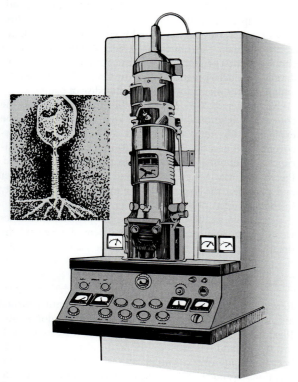

Fig. 3.4 The electron microscope has made possible the study of viruses, which cannot be seen with other microscopes.

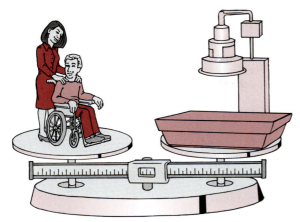

Fig. 3.5 Although technologic advances in radiography have been monumental, care provided by human beings is equally important in delivering the highest quality of care possible.

Alzheimer disease has prompted extensive research; its cause remains elusive, and treatment, though still in its infancy, is progressing. The prevention and treatment of human immunodeficiency viral (HIV) infection and acquired immunodeficiency syndrome (AIDS) have increased in importance as both conditions have become global.

Biotechnology has opened frontiers in treatment that were unimagined when this text was first published. Increasing numbers of surgeries and other interventional procedures are being made obsolete by the introduction of biotechnology into mainstream health care. Robotic surgery permits more precise incisions and excisions than ever before possible. Carefully guided by three-dimensional video, the surgeon probes deep into the body with a small computer-assisted *hand*. Robotic surgery is leading the way to improved patient outcomes when compared with open and even laparoscopic surgery. Advantages of robotic surgery include less blood loss, faster recovery for the patient, and fewer overall complications. It may be used for heart surgery, urinary system procedures, and prostate surgery.

The electrical conduction system of the heart has now been mapped. Patients with tachycardia or atrial fibrillation benefit from ablation procedures that use radiofrequency catheters to burn away errant pathways and permanently restore normal heart rate and rhythm.

The International Space Station is staffed full time and, as a result, new and ongoing research is taking place in the fields of human physiology and pharmacology that will have extensive applications back here on earth.

HEALTH AND DISEASE

No discussion of health care delivery would be complete without examining the status of health and disease. These conditions affect your patients. These will be the main causes of your patients' death. As a professional health care provider, you will want to be very familiar with your patients and their afflictions.

The World Health Organization defines **health** as "a state of complete physical, mental, and social well-being, and not merely the absence of disease or infirmity." Sheldon defines **disease** as "the pattern of response of a living organism to some form of injury"; he goes on to explain that disease "should be viewed as disordered function rather than only as altered structure."

Because measuring health status is a time-consuming, complicated, and often subjective process, we have continued to rely on data that indicate rates of **mortality** (death rate) and **morbidity** (occurrence of disease or conditions). It is apparent that Americans live long and have fewer acute episodes of illness than ever before, but we also have more chronic conditions than ever. Our population is affected by arthritis, chronic respiratory diseases, heart and circulatory problems, cancer, allergies, chronic digestive disorders, and alcohol and drug abuse.

Before moving on in this chapter, it must be noted that, at best, statistics are but a snapshot of a moment in time. Although all data in this chapter are accurate as of the date of publication, it is up to you, the radiography student, to remain current in your knowledge of health statistics by frequently visiting the web sites listed on this page.

Life Expectancy

Overall life expectancy in the United States is 78.6 years. The female-to-male difference in life expectancy is 5.0 years. Box 3.1 summarizes facts regarding life expectancy.

Mortality

Mortality statistics reveal much about life and death in the United States. The Centers for Disease Control and Prevention (CDC) through its National Center for Health Statistics (NCHS) gathers and publishes such data. The mission of the CDC is to promote health and the quality of life by preventing and controlling disease, injury, and disability. The primary sources of health statistics in this chapter are from CDC: www.cdc.gov and NCHS: www.cdc.gov/nchs.

The 10 leading causes of death in the United States (Box 3.2), including all races, both genders, and all ages, are listed. When reviewing this list, it should be noted that mortality rates are higher for men for *each* of the 10 leading causes of death.

BOX 3.1   Life Expectancy in the United States

National Center for Health Statistics. Please note that the Centers for Disease Control and Prevention uses the following terms to describe the four major population groups in the United States: *White, Black, Hispanic,* and *Native American.* The terms *Caucasian* and *African American* are not used.

Life Expectancy at Birth, in Years

Life expectancy by gender:
  All Males 76.1
  All Females 81.1
Life expectancy by race:
  Hispanic 82.8
  White 78.9
  Black 74.6
Life expectancy by race and gender:
  Hispanic female 84.0
  White female: 81.1
  Hispanic male: 79.0
  Black female: 78.4
  White male: 76.7
  Black male: 72.3
Life expectancy at age 65:
  All Americans: an additional 19.4 years
  All women: an additional 20.0 years
  All men: an additional 18.0 years

Centers for Disease Control and Prevention. Available at http://www.cdc.gov

BOX 3.2   The 10 Leading Causes of Death in the United States

1. Heart disease
2. Cancer
3. Unintentional injury (accidents, including motor vehicle fatalities)
4. Chronic lower respiratory diseases
5. Cerebrovascular diseases (stroke)
6. Alzheimer disease
7. Diabetes
8. Influenza and pneumonia
9. Kidney disease
10. Suicide

Centers for Disease Control and Prevention. Available at http://www.cdc.gov

Box 3.3 provides the five leading causes of death by age group. These lists seldom change in content but, because treatments improve, the population ages, and lifestyles alter, the causes of death sometime change in ranking. Hence, you should visit the above web sites annually.

Although death from some causes has decreased (e.g., the HIV mortality rate has declined by more than 70% since 1995 and is no longer among the top 15 causes of death), the aging of the population has witnessed an increase in the number of deaths from:

Alzheimer disease
Kidney disease
Hypertension
Parkinson disease

Causes of Death by Gender

Women: the number of deaths from breast cancer exceeds 40,000 annually.
Maternal mortality (i.e., death from complications of pregnancy, childbirth, and the postpartum period) is nearly 8 deaths in 100,000 live births.
Men: the number of deaths from prostate cancer exceeds 30,000 annually.

Causes of Death by Race

White
Heart disease
Cancer
Chronic lower respiratory diseases
Black
Heart disease
Cancer
Cerebrovascular diseases (stroke)
Hispanic
Cancer
Heart disease
Unintentional injury (accidents, including motor vehicle fatalities)

Specific Causes of Death

Firearm Deaths
White: 2.6 per 100,000 persons
Hispanic: 4.9 per 100,000 persons
Black: 20.9 per 100,000 persons
Note: Persons aged 15 to 34 years have the largest number of deaths from firearms.

Drugs
Death rate overall: 16.3 per 100,000 persons
Death rate among women: 11.3 per 100,000 persons
Death rate among men: 18.7 per 100,000 persons

BOX 3.3   The Five Leading Causes of Death in the United States by Age Group

Younger than 1 Year
Congenital anomalies
Short gestation
SIDS (sudden infant death syndrome)
Maternal pregnancy complications
Unintentional injury (accidents, including motor vehicle fatalities)

Ages 1–4 Years
Unintentional injury (accidents, including motor vehicle fatalities)
Congenital anomalies
Malignant neoplasms
Homicide
Heart disease

Ages 5–9 Years
Unintentional injury (accidents, including motor vehicle fatalities)
Malignant neoplasms
Congenital anomalies
Homicide
Heart disease

Ages 10–14 Years
Unintentional injury (accidents, including motor vehicle fatalities)
Suicide
Malignant neoplasms
Homicide
Congenital anomalies

Ages 15–24 Years
Unintentional injury (accidents, including motor vehicle fatalities)
Suicide
Homicide
Malignant neoplasms
Heart disease

Ages 25–34 Years
Unintentional injury (accidents, including motor vehicle fatalities)
Suicide
Homicide
Malignant neoplasms
Heart disease

Ages 35–44 Years
Unintentional injury (accidents, including motor vehicle fatalities)
Malignant neoplasms
Heart disease
Suicide
Homicide

Ages 45–54 Years
Malignant neoplasms
Heart disease
Unintentional injury (accidents, including motor vehicle fatalities)
Suicide
Liver disease

Ages 55–64 Years
Malignant neoplasms
Heart disease
Unintentional injury (accidents, including motor vehicle fatalities)
Chronic lower respiratory disease
Diabetes

Ages 65 Years and Older
Heart disease
Malignant neoplasms
Chronic lower respiratory disease
Cerebrovascular diseases (stroke)
Alzheimer disease

Centers for Disease Control and Prevention. Available at http://www.cdc.gov

Note: In states that have legalized recreational marijuana, fatalities in motor vehicle accidents have tripled because of driving under the influence of marijuana.

Alcohol
Death rate is approximately 9.6 per 100,000 persons.
Death rate among men is 3.5 times higher than the death rate for women.

Infant Mortality
Death rate is just below 7 deaths per 1000 live births, the lowest rate ever recorded in the United States.

Morbidity

In addition to death, morbidity takes its toll. Previously defined as the rate of occurrence of diseases or conditions, the following are the primary causes of disablement, medical intervention, health care expenditures, and overall lack of wellness in the United States:

Obesity (including close to 17% of children diagnosed as obese, climbing nearly 2% per year)

Mental and emotional disorders, including alcohol and drug abuse

Diseases of the cardiovascular system

Alzheimer disease

Asthma

Arthritis

Hypertension

Influenza

Food-borne illnesses

Epilepsy

Cerebral palsy

Multiple sclerosis

Parkinson disease

Muscular dystrophy

Hearing and visual impairments

Diabetes

Cancer

Select Morbidity by Race and Gender (ages 20 years and older)

Obesity
Black women: 56%
Hispanic women: 45%
Hispanic men: 39%
Black men: 37%
White women: 36%
White men: 34%

Hypertension
Black women: 44%
Black men: 40%
White women: 34%
White men: 34%
Hispanic women: 23%
Hispanic men: 20%

Smokers (ages 18 years and older)
Hispanic women: 23%
Black men: 21%
White men: 19%
White women: 17%
Black women: 14%
Hispanic men: 7%

Overall Health Reported as Fair or Poor
Black: 13.6%
Hispanic: 10.4%
White: 9.5%

Emerging Infectious Diseases

Modern medicine has triumphantly eradicated smallpox and is nearing the elimination of polio. Other diseases targeted for worldwide eradication, severe limitation, or elimination by region include guinea worm, onchocerciasis, syphilis, rabies, measles, tuberculosis, and leprosy.

However, the threat from emerging and reemerging infectious diseases has become the leading cause of death and disability worldwide (Box 3.4). Dramatic changes in society, technology, and the environment, as well as a diminished effectiveness of some approaches to disease control, have allowed this development to occur.

The term **emerging infectious diseases** refers to diseases of infectious origin whose incidence in human beings has either increased within the past 2 decades or threatens to increase in the near future. Such diseases increasingly threaten public health and substantially increase the cost of health care. Infectious diseases account for 25% of all visits to physicians each year, and antimicrobial agents are the second most frequently prescribed class of drugs in the United States. For example, childhood ear infections are the leading cause of visits to pediatricians, and the incidence of visits for such infections has increased by 150%. Direct and indirect costs of infectious diseases exceed $120 billion.

Emerging infections are especially serious in people with lowered immunity, such as those who are HIV positive, those receiving immunosuppressive chemotherapy, and those who have received transplanted organs; these are all growing populations. Other large groups affected by this threat are older adults, those cared for in institutions, people with inadequate access to health care, and more than 11 million children in day care centers.

BOX 3.4   Emerging Infectious Diseases Worldwide

Anthrax infections (bioterrorism)
Coccidioidomycosis
Cryptosporidiosis
Drug-resistant *Mycobacterium tuberculosis*
Drug-resistant pneumococcal disease
Drug-resistant *Staphylococcus aureus*
Escherichia coli O 157:H7 disease
Hantavirus pulmonary syndrome
HIV/AIDS—global
Influenza A, Beijing, 32, 92
Vancomycin-resistant enterococcal infections
West Nile fever

Centers for Disease Control and Prevention. Available at http://www.cdc.gov

Disease emergence can be related to many factors. Newly emergent infectious diseases may result from changes in or the evolution of existing organisms; known diseases may spread to new geographic areas or human populations; or previously unrecognized infections may appear in people living or working in areas undergoing ecologic changes (e.g., deforestation, reforestation) that increase human exposure to insects, animals, or environmental sources that may harbor new or unusual infectious agents. Global travel increases the possibility of spreading a disease that otherwise may have remained isolated. The threat of bioterrorism further complicates the issue.

Furthermore, infectious diseases may reemerge because of either the development of antimicrobial resistance in existing agents (e.g., gonorrhea, malaria, pneumococci) or breakdowns in public health measures for previously controlled infections (e.g., cholera, tuberculosis, pertussis). Such infections can affect people in geographically widespread areas regardless of lifestyle, cultural or ethnic background, or socioeconomic status.

It is important for the health care professional to understand two key terms when discussing infectious diseases—epidemic and pandemic. An **epidemic** is a widespread infectious disease within a given geographic area. A **pandemic** is an infectious disease of global proportions. Health care leaders and researchers are trying to contain increasing numbers of emerging infectious diseases to prevent pandemics.

Surveillance of infectious diseases in the United States depends on voluntary collaboration among the CDC and state and local health departments, which in turn depend on reporting by health care professionals. Such reporting is frequently incomplete.

The CDC has established the following goals for dealing with the threat of emerging infectious diseases:
- Goal 1: Detect, promptly investigate, and monitor emerging pathogens, the diseases they cause, and the factors that influence their emergence.
- Goal 2: Integrate laboratory science and epidemiology to optimize public health practice.
- Goal 3: Enhance communication of public health information about emerging diseases and ensure prompt implementation of prevention strategies.
- Goal 4: Strengthen local, state, and federal public health infrastructures to support surveillance and to implement prevention and control programs.

Implementation of these goals and their accompanying objectives are relevant to health care delivery and its reform. Relevant issues include prolonged hospitalization as a result of health care–acquired infections, increased morbidity and treatment costs resulting from antimicrobial drug resistance, and excessive burdens placed on public and private health care delivery facilities because of community-wide outbreaks of foodborne and waterborne infections.

SOCIAL FORCES THAT AFFECT HEALTH CARE

As a radiologic technologist, you are part of a larger health care system that, in some way, touches the lives of everyone. The technologic advances alone have been dramatic. These improvements—coupled with a deeper understanding of the human being at the focus of our care—provide the basis for the continual evolution of health care delivery.

Economic and social forces not in existence in centuries past deeply affect today's health care system. As a key member of the health care team, you, too, are influenced. The quality of the care you provide is profoundly determined by the environment in which you practice and by your professional self-image. Chapter 6 discusses in detail the values you can add to the services you provide. Such values enhance not only the patient's experience but also your self-image. The challenges are many; consequently, the opportunities for professional growth are plentiful. However, radiologic technologists must have an understanding of the continually changing health care climate.

The aging of the population and increasing health care costs are key forces that are greatly changing health care delivery. Although diagnostic imaging will continue to play a prominent role in health care, its exact shape will continue to evolve. You have chosen a field of study that has a bright future but that will certainly have its peaks and valleys over time. The venues in which radiologic technologists practice continue to change, and the job market fluctuates constantly. However, radiologic technology will continue to be one of the fastest-growing occupations in the coming decades. Within the profession, individual fields will grow even faster than others, such as education and all forms of scanning and digital imaging.

Your patients and employers will expect and require the best of your talents and skills. They require a strong command of both the technical aspects of radiologic technology and the high-touch aspects of patient care and service. More work must be done with fewer caregivers when dealing with the realities of health care financing. You will also need a working knowledge of health care delivery issues.

ETHICAL ISSUES

The advances in research and technology in medicine have prompted disagreement about ethical issues as never before. With all of its hope and ability to enhance the quality of life, health care has also raised questions that society must answer. Professionals and private citizens alike debate issues such as the patient's right to privacy and confidentiality of information. This topic has become particularly sensitive since the outbreak of AIDS. Animal rights advocates decry the use of laboratory animals in medical experiments; other groups question whether new drugs are made available to human beings too soon or not soon enough.

Health care–related issues dominate the medical, religious, and political arenas. The elusive question of when life begins has yet to be answered by either science or the courts. At the other end of the life cycle is the debate over when life ends. Accompanying these controversies are the issues of abortion, active euthanasia (assisted suicide), passive euthanasia, and the right to die.

In vitro fertilization is a reality as is surrogate motherhood. Genetic engineering carries with it the hope for the elimination of inherited diseases, as well as the specter of selecting which offspring to carry to term. Ultimately, the most sensitive ethical issue may be the rationing of health care.

Concern about long-term care for an aging population becomes greater with each passing year. As the twenty-first century unfolds, more than 10 million older adults need care, and more than 3 million are in institutions with that number growing annually. By the year 2025, half of all older Americans will be 75 years of age or older. Even now, more than two thirds of those in nursing homes have some form of cognitive disorder such as Alzheimer disease. Most of the cost of long-term care is paid for by the nursing home residents, their families, or both; depletion of life savings in a very short period is not unusual. Some underwriters offer a form of long-term care insurance coverage, and the government is examining its role in funding such care.

Because of the sheer increase in the number of citizens in this age group, home care is on a steady increase. Home health care products cover simple hygiene, as well as complex medical technology. In some areas, physicians and dentists make house calls. Mobile radiography services provide diagnostic testing in the community. Visiting nurses make their daily rounds in nearly every locale.

Serious ethical issues will likely be resolved by the judicial system long before science provides solutions. Indeed, science may not be able to answer the moral questions that have been raised. Discussions of these and other ethical controversies of the health care delivery system have an important place in your education.

Radiologic technologists must remember that these are times that require immense flexibility in dealing with all types of patients of all ages and in various clinical situations. It is a time of constant change and almost unlimited opportunity for professional challenge and personal growth.

ECONOMIC FORCES THAT AFFECT HEALTH CARE

Cost is a major issue in the status of health care delivery. Health care expenditures are nearing 20% of the gross domestic product (GDP) of the United States; this figure amounts to $3.5 trillion annually (Box 3.5).

The question of paying for health care is answered by examining the sources of such funding.

Health Spending by Major Sources of Funds

Private health insurance: 34%
Medicare: 20%
Medicaid: 17%
Out of pocket: 11%
Other: 18%

We spend more of our GDP on health care than any other nation in the world, primarily because of the costs of salaries and benefits for health care professionals and the availability of medical technology and care nearly everywhere. The cost of health care in the United States has generally increased faster than the prevailing rate of inflation for more than 4 decades. Those who pay most of the nation's medical bills are the federal and state governments and private insurance companies. Historically, rates were set by the providers of health care (e.g., hospitals, physicians), and then third-party payers (e.g., insurance companies, the government) reimbursed the providers

---

BOX 3.5   Health Care Spending by Type of Service or Product

Hospital care: 32%
Physician and clinical services: 20%
Prescription drugs: 10%
Other Health, residential, and personal care services: 5% (schools, community health, ambulance, and so on)
Nursing care facilities and continuing care retirement communities: 5%
Dental services: 4%
Other professional services: 3% (rehabilitation, physical therapy, occupational therapy, and so on)
Home health care: 3%
Durable medical equipment: 2% (eyeglasses, hearing aids, and so on)
Other nondurable medical products: 2% (over the counter meds, bandages, and so on)
Other: 14%

From National Health Expenditure Data. http://www.cms.gov

for that amount. With rising costs, this system could not continue.

A **prospective payment system** (PPS) is now in place. Under this structure, the government pays medical bills for older adults (Medicare) and the needy (Medicaid) based on diagnostic-related groups (DRGs). The cost for providing services, which is determined ahead of time by the government, is based on the admitting diagnosis. Hospitals are pressed to provide the service at or below the level of payment. If costs exceed the predetermined amount, the hospital must absorb those costs. If care is provided at a lower cost, the hospital may keep the extra payment.

Most third-party payers now incorporate some form of prospective payment or negotiated fees as part of their contract for payment. Many patients are members of **health maintenance organizations** (HMOs) that offer, for a monthly fee, all necessary medical care at no additional charge. Some HMOs own their own hospitals or contract with others for the care of their members. Others are members of preferred provider organizations (PPOs) that negotiate lower fees with the patient's insurer. This entire system has forced hospitals to reduce overhead, examine cost schedules, and limit unnecessary medical care and services. The result has been a decline in the use of expensive inpatient services and a greater use of cost-effective outpatient facilities. This change has greatly affected hospitals that historically relied on inpatient revenues. Most have had to realign their services with patient needs and payer requirements.

The political arena is congested with debate about the role of Medicare and the federal government overall in health care financing. The effect on the patients you serve can be profound. The older patient may be concerned that Medicare will not pay the entire bill. Early discharge from the hospital may be indicated because of limits on coverage for a given medical condition. Other patients have experienced medical insurance premiums rising 10% to 20% each year. Increased deductibles on insurance policies, whether they are individual or group plans, transfer more of the actual cost of care directly onto the patient. Such costs affect each patient as never before. The Affordable Care Act was an attempt at making more insurance available to more people by mandating the purchase of health insurance, either from private insurers or public providers. The law was controversial; the effect on insurance and health care costs is debatable.

Trying to hold the line on health care costs is not easy. Just as some price controls are put into place, other factors cause fees to rise. Salaries, the highest single cost in health care, must be kept at competitive levels to attract and retain excellent clinicians. In fact, labor costs account for more than 70% of the average hospital's budget. Labor shortages in some areas of health care have placed upward pressure on salaries. New technologies carry with them high price tags; some estimate that the latest technology adds 50% to the patient's bill for each day in the hospital. Supplies for hospitals are costly, and new services must be offered to attract and serve patients. Finally, as the population ages and the majority of patients are older than 75 years of age, the medical care required increases because of a higher incidence of disability and chronic disease. Chronic disease consumes more than 80% of the health care resources. Approximately 33% of the average American's lifetime health spending occurs during the final year of life, with almost half that amount spent in the last 2 months of life; along with this goes the total nation's health bill. In addition to fewer people in the workforce to pay into government programs and group insurance, these factors are wreaking havoc with the delivery of health care.

No single solution to the problem of health care cost reimbursement exists. Hospitals and health care workers must do all they can to control costs. The question of who pays the bill must be answered. Many people carry no insurance or are not covered at their place of employment. The cost of medical care for them is absorbed by the hospital system or Medicaid. Furthermore, such individuals many times do not seek care at all, thus worsening their existing medical conditions, which ultimately results in higher costs for more serious problems. However, if employers are forced to cover all employees under group insurance, then a serious financial strain is placed on their ability to compete with larger companies with greater resources or with foreign companies who carry no such burden. If all citizens were covered under a single-payer form of national health insurance, as is proposed by some, tax rates would skyrocket.

Another factor that affects the cost of health care is the practice of defensive medicine. **Defensive medicine** can be defined as any waste of resources (i.e., net excess of costs over benefits) that results from physicians changing their patterns of practice in response to the threat of malpractice liability (McLennan and Meyer, 1989). In a society that goes to court over almost anything, alleged medical malpractice is a high-visibility target. Defensive medicine, coupled with the dramatically increased cost of malpractice insurance premiums for physicians and hospitals alike, adds to the cost of providing services. Quality assurance has become a constant partner in the practice of medicine. Nevertheless, the overall cost is something that must be addressed sooner or later.

There seems to be no easy answer. Obviously, you as a health care worker will be affected by the system in which you work, both as an employee and as a patient. Your understanding of and involvement in the professional and political issues that affect your chosen career are vital. Keep abreast of these issues by maintaining membership and actively participating in your professional organizations.

NEED FOR HEALTH CARE MANAGEMENT

One of the best ways of holding down health care costs and improving the quality of life is the practice of preventive medicine. The impetus comes from business, which has seen rising medical care expenses reduce profits and inhibit the ability to compete in a global economy. Whether by directly paying expenses, having high absenteeism, or experiencing lower productivity, the business world has come to realize that managing the health of employees also allows it to maximize profits and benefits.

Companies report that most health care expenditures are directly connected to the lifestyle of their employees. According to the CDC, more than half of early deaths are attributable to lifestyle. Box 3.6 correlates the risk

---

BOX 3.6   Risk Factors and Primary Causes of Death

Heart Disease
Sedentary lifestyle
Cigarette smoking
Hypertension
Obesity
Diabetes
High cholesterol
Cancer
Cigarette smoking
Positive stool occult blood
Failure to perform breast self-examination
Failure to have Papanicolaou tests (Pap smears)

Cerebrovascular Disease
Cigarette smoking
Hypertension
High cholesterol

Accidents
Failure to use seat belts
High alcohol use

Chronic Lower Respiratory Disease
Cigarette smoking

Centers for Disease Control and Prevention. Available at http://www.cdc.gov

---

factors with the top five causes of death. Sedentary lifestyle, not using seat belts, smoking, alcohol, and diet play key roles in more than 70% of the cases for each cause of death.

PREVENTIVE MEDICINE

If most causes of disease, disability, and even death are directly related to lifestyle, then it is clear that wellness and health care costs can be managed. More and more employers now offer some form of wellness program to employees. These offers may take the form of in-house education and activities or memberships at local health and fitness facilities. Screening employees for high blood pressure, elevated cholesterol, abnormal glucose levels, and threatening lifestyle habits is commonplace. Counseling is provided in such areas as smoking cessation, proper nutrition, fitness, weight control, and stress management. Emphasis on prevention rather than medical intervention is the key to a healthy lifestyle, as well as to a healthy medical delivery system. An indication of the potential savings is reflected in the fact that smoking-related illnesses alone cost the health care system (i.e., taxpayers, insurance premium payers) more than $65 billion annually. If tobacco use in the United States stopped entirely, an estimated 390,000 fewer Americans would die before their time each year. If alcohol were never carelessly used, approximately 100,000 fewer people would die from unnecessary illness and injury. AIDS—another almost entirely preventable disease—costs in excess of $13 billion annually to treat.

Two lifestyle factors that are related to health are **smoking** and **diet**. Many states have passed clean indoor air laws that prohibit or severely limit smoking in public places. In addition to the increased risk to the smoker, the effect on nonsmokers is serious. Secondhand smoke greatly increases the occurrence of cancer, heart disease, and lung illnesses, and it also aggravates preexisting conditions. Approximately 38 million American smokers who quit before they reach the 50 years of age can reduce their risk of dying in the next 15 years by half; the risk of heart disease and lung cancer returns to the level of a nonsmoker in 5 to 10 years. Furthermore, data indicate that those who smoke spend nearly $1000 more per year for medical care. In view of its link to virtually every major illness, it is surprising that 50 million people still smoke. However, a rapidly changing health care delivery system that is based on preventive care may change that figure in the coming years.

Box 3.7 summarizes the dietary guidelines from the These guidelines are published every five years, so you will want to revisit this document on a regular basis. United States Departments of Agriculture and Health and Human Services.

BOX 3.7   Dietary Guidelines

Eat a variety of foods.

Maintain an ideal weight.

Consume less than 10 percent of calories per day from saturated fats.

Limit cholesterol intake.

Increase protein intake including seafood, lean meats and poultry, eggs, legumes (beans and peas), and nuts, seeds, and soy products.

Consume less than 2,300 milligrams (mg) per day of sodium.

Increase consumption of fruits, vegetables, and whole grains.

- If alcohol is consumed, it should be consumed in moderation—up to one drink per day for women and up to two drinks per day for men—and only by adults of legal drinking age.

Consume less than 10 percent of calories per day from added sugars.

Except for young children, substitute low-fat and nonfat milk for whole milk and low-fat dairy products for high-fat dairy products.

Dietary Guidelines for Americans, 2015–2020

Chemicals, food additives, salt, sugar, and alcohol by themselves, perhaps, should not cause alarm. However, when you consider the combined effects of these factors, how diet mismanagement leads to major health problems is easy to understand.

Preventable conditions could save the nation billions of dollars at a time when fewer workers are available to pay the bills for expensive diagnoses and treatments. Injuries cost more than $100 billion annually, cancer costs more than $70 billion, and cardiovascular disease costs more than $135 billion.

Good health comes from reducing unnecessary suffering, illness, and disability; it stresses improved quality of life and a sense of well-being. Renewed efforts on all fronts will help our nation achieve its goals. Ultimately, individual lifestyle choices will be the determining factor. For a student who is contemplating a career in health care, a healthy lifestyle will not only result in a happier, more productive education and working life, but it will also set an example for patients and coworkers.

HEALTH CARE SYSTEM

Our health care system is laden with the values of our society. In the United States, our health care system has many components as described by Torrens:

1. Public health and preventive medicine
2. Emergency medical care
3. Simple, nonemergency, ambulatory patient care
4. Complex, ambulatory patient care
5. Simple, inpatient hospital care
6. Complex, inpatient hospital care
7. Long-term, continuing care and rehabilitation
8. Care for social, emotional, and developmental problems
9. Transportation
10. Financial compensations for disability

Even with the necessary elements, such a system is useless unless the patient has the desire and confidence to use it. The patient's attitude is often determined by the demeanor and attitude of the health care provider. As a radiologic technologist, you have the opportunity to educate your patients about a particular radiologic examination and to inform them of other health care services, how they can be reached, and the value of the services. You can help educate people about their own health care and show them how to become more directly responsible for their lives and health; this approach is an example of total patient care and value-added service.

Traditionally, health care has been practiced in hospitals that offer a full range of services, from diagnostic testing to surgery and drug therapy. The emphasis has been on medical intervention. However, hospitals, along with businesses, are now heavily involved in wellness programs. They have also modified their traditional services to reflect a changing market. Outpatient clinics account for more diagnostic testing and simple treatment and cost far less than being admitted to a hospital emergency department. Many forms of surgery are performed on an outpatient basis. The graduate radiologic technologist of the near future will likely practice in an urgent care clinic, a group physicians imaging center, or an ambulatory care institution in addition to a conventional acute care hospital.

Hospitals respect the rights of their primary customer—the patient. It is recognized that patients are not just creatures to whom we are *doing things*; they are dignified individuals with emotions and feelings, likes and dislikes. In support of this attitude, the American Hospital Association adopted the *Patient's Bill of Rights*.

The health care system in the United States is in a constant state of change as the twenty-first century evolves. Most of the issues presented in this chapter are being debated daily. Some will be resolved, and others will not. Many will be decided by the US Congress and ruled on by the judiciary. Diagnostic procedures and methods of patient care are evolving as quickly as researchers can verify results. Health care delivery is changing faster than textbooks can be revised. Many of today's common treatments and procedures were at one time subject to ridicule, skepticism, and evaluation. Furthermore, approximately 85% of the technology in a hospital today had not been invented 10 years ago.

Radiologic technologists must draw on their years of education and experience to keep an open mind to the social and technologic changes as new methods of patient care and treatment enter the health care arena. It is hoped that all forms of medicine—preventive, interventional, and alternative—will come together for the benefit of all patients. You have chosen a career that can help fulfill this hope.

BEGINNING OF YOUR CHALLENGE

The status of health care delivery in no small part depends on you. Your work ethic, dedication to excellence, and unwillingness to provide anything but the best patient care and quality service are of paramount importance.

As you begin your clinical education, immediately establish your reputation. Work hard and do more than is expected; your patients and potential employers will take notice. Your patients will reward you with their gratitude, spoken or unspoken. Your potential employers, who are the clinical supervisors and department heads in radiology, begin making hiring decisions very early in the educational process; their reward may well be your first job in radiography. Most important, your dedication to excellence and hard work will build your self-esteem and confidence.

The challenge is there for those who want to meet it. As the web of health care delivery becomes more tangled, it becomes more important for each health care worker to realize the important roles that all members of the team play. Professionalism should not be your goal; rather, professionalism is the path to follow toward your other goals. It is something to be practiced each and every day. True professionals rise to meet the challenges. They treat patients as guests and send them on their way feeling as if each one was the most important person cared for that day.

You are beginning a vitally important educational process. You are not *in training* for anything. Training tells you how to do something, but education tells you why you are doing it. Learning the technology that comprises radiography is essential to your practice. Dealing with patients and their families—and your coworkers—with human warmth, understanding, and genuine caring will be vital to your satisfaction and the success of your career. Establishing good study habits and clinical behavior right from the start will help you greatly when the time comes to enter the job market.

CONCLUSION

The history of medicine and the evolution of health care delivery are being recorded even as you begin your studies in radiologic technology. Medicine is advancing at a rapid pace. The possibilities for improvements in the quality and longevity of life are only as limited as the dreams and hard work of all involved in health care, including you in your studies and lifestyle choices.

The author of this book hopes that this text will help you get off to a good start, whether you are studying to make a career choice or beginning your radiography education. Thousands before you have used this book to begin their journey. Return to it again and again for reference or review; use it to explain to friends and family what it is you are studying to become; recruit new student radiologic technologists—the future of our profession—by sharing this book with them.

This is indeed the beginning of your challenge. You have many months of exciting work ahead of you. Do more than is required during your educational process, and you will meet with a degree of success that you can only imagine today.

QUESTIONS FOR DISCUSSION AND CRITICAL THINKING

1. Discuss some of the basic health care practices from ancient times and compare them with today's practice of health care.
2. Discuss the advances in medicine that occurred in the Renaissance and determine which are still relevant today.
3. Explain what you believe to be the top 10 advances in health care from the eighteenth, nineteenth, twentieth, and twenty-first centuries. Defend your choices.
4. Discuss the causes of death by age group and possible prevention of those deaths.
5. Review causes of death by race and gender. Attempt to correlate them to socioeconomics, education, availability of care, and so on.
6. Review morbidity and discuss preventive measures.
7. Compare pandemic with epidemic. Describe the importance of understanding these terms by the radiographer.
8. Discuss and debate the role of private insurers and the federal government (taxpayers) in the payment for health care services.
9. Discuss the role of preventive medicine in health care.

BIBLIOGRAPHY

Bettman O. *A pictorial history of medicine.* Springfield, IL: Charles C. Thomas; 1979. Available from, http://www.cdc.gov.

Centers for Disease Control and Prevention. Available at http://www.cdc.gov.

Centers for Medicare and Medicaid Services. Available at www.cms.gov.

Green J. *Medical history for students.* Springfield, IL: Charles C. Thomas; 1968.

Lyons AS, Petrucelli RJ. *Medicine: an illustrated history.* New York: Harry Abrams; 1978.

Major R: *A history of medicine,* vol 1, Springfield, IL, 1954, Charles C. Thomas.

McLennan K, Meyer J. *Care and cost: current issues in health policy.* Boulder, CO: Westview Press; 1989.

Torrens PR. *The American health system issues and problems.* St. Louis: Mosby; 1978.

Sheldon H. *Boyd's introduction to the study of disease.* Philadelphia: LWW; 1992.

Senate United States Departments of Agriculture and Health and Human Services. Dietary Guidelines for Americans, ed. 8; 2015.

4

Radiology: *A Historic Perspective*

OBJECTIVES

On completion of this chapter, you should be able to:
- List the pioneers in radiology and describe their contributions to the field.
- Describe the events leading to the discovery of x-rays.
- Give a short history of Wilhelm Conrad Roentgen.
- Describe the works of Marie and Pierre Curie in radioactivity.
- List the events leading to the development of nuclear medicine.
- Describe the modern radiology department, including equipment, specialized tasks, and staff development through continuing education.

OUTLINE

Pioneers of Radiology
  Wilhelm Roentgen
Early Days in the Discovery
Advanced Experimentation With Roentgen Rays

Nuclear Radiology
Modern Digital Radiography
Conclusion

KEY TERMS

algorithms
Anna Bertha Roentgen
barium platinocyanide
computer memory
computed tomography
cyclotron

diagnostic medical sonography
digital radiography
fluoroscopy
interventional radiology
Johann Wilhelm Hittorf
radioactivity

microprocessor speed
nuclear radiology
magnetic resonance imaging
Thomas Edison
Wilhelm Conrad Roentgen
William Crookes

Few discoveries have so profoundly affected the world as the discovery of the x-ray. This development has changed almost every aspect of medical practice. However, the diagnosis and treatment of disease is not the only area influenced by this discovery. Other uses have also had a dramatic effect on the way we live and work and include, for example, providing security at airports, developing improved strains of grain, controlling some kinds of insects, detecting flaws in industrial materials and equipment, identifying counterfeit art, and, recently, irradiating food to extend its shelf life.

PIONEERS OF RADIOLOGY

The development of radiology is, in large measure, a story of the development of technical hardware. The work of early scientists and craftsmen made possible the production of x-rays. Evidence of experimentation with the chemical, as well as the physical properties of matter, has been found as early as the first century AD. Archimedes, for example, explained the reaction of solids when they are placed in liquids. Democritus described materials as being composed of ultimate particles, and Thales discovered some of the effects of electricity.

More recently, three specific aspects of physical science helped pave the way for the discovery of x-rays—electricity, vacuums, and image-recording materials. Evangelista Torricelli produced the first-recognized vacuum when he invented a barometer in 1643. In 1646, through many hours of scientific experiments, Otto van Guericke invented an air pump that was capable of removing air from a vessel or tube. This experiment was repeated in 1659 by Robert Boyle and in 1865 by Herman Sprengel. Their techniques considerably improved the amount of evacuation, thus making better vacuum tubes available for further experimentation by other scientists.

From the seventeenth century forward, the main interest of scientists seemed to be experimentation with electricity. William Gilbert of England was one of the first to extensively study electricity and magnetism. He was also noted for inventing a primitive electroscope. Robert Boyle's experiments with electricity earned him a place among the serious investigators. Most such scientists had to build their own equipment. Isaac Newton built and improved the static generator. Charles du Fay, working with glass, silk, and paper, distinguished two different kinds of electricity.

Abbé Jean-Antoine Nollet made a significant improvement in the electroscope, a vessel for discharging electricity under vacuum conditions. The electroscope was a forerunner of the x-ray tube. Of course, Benjamin Franklin conducted many electrical experiments and should be mentioned in any discussion of the pioneers in electricity. William Watson demonstrated a current of electricity by transmitting electricity from a Leyden jar through wires and a vacuum tube.

While conducting experiments with electrical discharges, William Morgan noticed the difference in color of partially evacuated tubes. He noted that when a tube cracked and some air leaked in, the amount of air in the tube determined the coloration.

In 1831, Michael Faraday induced an electric current by moving a magnet in and out of a coil. From this experiment evolved the concept of electromagnetic induction, which led to the production of better generators and transformers and high voltages for use in evacuated tubes. The most significant improvement on induction coils was made by Heinrich Daniel Ruhmkorff of Paris.

Johann Wilhelm Hittorf conducted several experiments with cathode rays, which are streams of electrons emitted from the surface of a cathode. William Crookes furthered the study of cathode rays and demonstrated that matter was emitted from the cathode with enough energy to rotate a wheel placed within a tube. Hittorf's works were repeated and further developed by Crookes. Philipp Lenard furthered the investigation of the cathode rays. He found that cathode rays could penetrate thin metal and would project a few centimeters into the air. Lenard did a tremendous amount of research with cathode rays and determined their energies by measuring the amount of penetration. He also studied the deflection of rays as a result of magnetic fields.

William Goodspeed produced a radiograph in 1890. However, his achievement was recognized only in retrospect and after the discovery of x-rays by Wilhelm Conrad Roentgen; Goodspeed was not credited with the discovery of x-rays.

The image-recording materials (i.e., the photographic recording techniques) were very important to the investigators of the cathode rays. The first photographic copy of written material was produced by Johann Heinrich Schulze in 1727. This technique was tested further and greatly improved in later years. In 1871, Richard Leach Maddox produced a film with a gelatin silver bromide emulsion that later became the basic component for film. In 1884, George Eastman produced and patented roll-paper film. With this significant improvement of image-recording material and the improvement in the cathode ray tube, the basis for twentieth century radiography was established.

Wilhelm Roentgen

Wilhelm Conrad Roentgen was born on March 27, 1845, in Lennep, a small town near the Rhine River in Germany (Fig. 4.1, *A*). He was the only child of Friedrich Conrad Roentgen, a textile merchant whose ancestors had lived in or near Lennep for several generations. Wilhelm Roentgen married Bertha Ludwig in 1872 (Fig. 4.1, *B*), and in 1888, he was offered employment at the University of Wurzburg. He readily accepted the offer, knowing of the university's new physics institute and its impressive facilities. Roentgen was elected rector at the university, although he continued to work in the physics department and on his personal research projects. He became interested in cathode ray experiments with the Crookes tube, which he worked with until his discovery of x-rays.

Discovery of X-Rays

On November 8, 1895, Wilhelm Roentgen discovered x-rays while working in his modest laboratory at the university. While operating a Crookes tube at high voltage in a darkened room, he noticed a piece of barium platinocyanide paper on a bench several feet from the Crookes tube. He observed a glowing or fluorescence of the barium platinocyanide after he passed a current through the tube for only a short period. Knowing the parameters of this particular experiment, Roentgen realized that the fluorescence was some kind of ray, rather than light or electricity, escaping the Crookes tube.

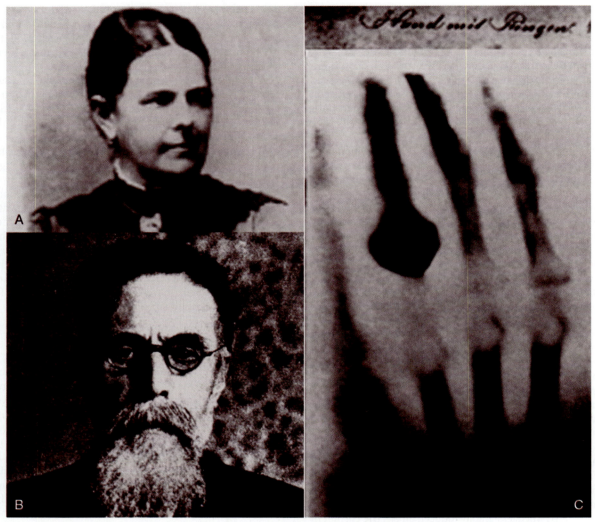

Fig. 4.1 **A,** Roentgen's wife, Anna Bertha Roentgen (1839–1919). **B,** Wilhelm C. Roentgen a few weeks before he died. **C,** Roentgen's first radiograph, showing his wife's hand and two rings on her finger. (From Glasser O: *Wilhelm Conrad Roentgen and the early history of the roentgen rays*, Springfield, IL, 1933, Charles C. Thomas.)

Roentgen proved that he had produced some type of x-ray (x being a mathematical symbol for an unknown quantity) by continuously producing the fluorescent effect of the barium platinocyanide. By performing several more tests with the mysterious rays he determined that the x-rays had a degree of penetrative power dependent on the density of the material.

On December 28, 1895, Roentgen submitted a report titled, "On a New Kind of Rays" to the Wurzburg Physico-Medical Society. He realized that this new type of ray could potentially have a medical use. Putting this thought into action, Roentgen discovered that by placing his hand between the tube and a piece of cardboard coated with barium platinocyanide, he could actually visualize the bones of his hand, thus demonstrating the primitive fluoroscopic screen. He knew he had discovered something that could revolutionize the world of science, but he still did not know whether his observations were correct. This prompted him to further test the cathode rays so that he could prove the validity of his previous experiments.

After several weeks of working in virtual seclusion, Roentgen proved that his previous work was, in fact, valid. He tried another experiment in which he convinced his wife, **Anna Bertha Roentgen**, to place her hand on a cassette loaded with a photographic plate upon which he directed the x-rays from the tube for approximately 15 minutes. Development of the plate proved again that Roentgen's experiments were successful. His observations were correct. The bones in his wife's hand, as well as the two rings on her finger, were clearly visible (Fig. 4.1, *C*). Roentgen had produced the world's first radiograph of a human.

Roentgen continued to study the effects of x-rays and presented his notes to different societies. In addition to many other awards and honors, Roentgen received the first Nobel Prize in Physics in 1901 in Stockholm and became a member of the Physical Society of Stockholm. In 1902, he received an invitation from the Carnegie Institute in Washington, DC, to use its laboratory for special experiments, but he did not accept the invitation. On February 10, 1923, Wilhelm Conrad Roentgen died in Munich, Germany.

EARLY DAYS IN THE DISCOVERY

The discovery of x-rays offered much hope in the discipline of science, but few discoveries have been so little understood by the general public. The nature of the rays is partly responsible for this. They cannot be sensed by sight, touch, taste, smell, or hearing. Consequently, explaining them is difficult. In 1895, when Wilhelm Roentgen discovered the as yet unknown rays and published his findings, the Western world immediately reacted and clamored for more information. Through newspapers, Thomas Alva Edison attempted to explain the nature of the rays to the citizens in the United States. However, no one fully understood the effects of radiation. This did not prevent entrepreneurs from taking risks and developing schemes for profit in the marketplace. Scientists and others produced a flurry of publications. Although some seriously attempted to explain the nature of the rays, others were vague, some were comic, and still others were clearly dishonest. In addition, jokes and cartoons were printed, as well as ludicrous advertisements appearing in newspapers (Fig. 4.2).

Circuses used x-rays for entertainment in guessing the contents of women's purses. Department stores and fairs offered bone portraits (Fig. 4.3). A manufacturing company produced lead underwear for modest women and men. England passed a law against opera glasses with x-ray vision. Some wealthy persons purchased x-ray units for their homes to entertain guests by imaging their skeletons with the fluoroscope (Fig. 4.4).

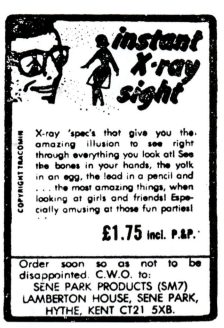

Fig. 4.2 An advertisement that capitalizes on the use of x-rays for profit. (From Eisenberg RL: *Radiology: an illustrated history*, St. Louis, 1992, Mosby.)

Abuses of these rays were rampant, and, in time, the latent effects on tissues began to show degenerating results. **Thomas Edison**, one of the most knowledgeable on the subject, took notice and questioned the effects of x-rays. He complained that his eyes were sore and red after working with a fluorescent tube. Although it was not clearly established that this was caused by x-rays, later reports coming from other workers in his laboratory confirmed a direct relationship between their injuries and x-ray exposure.

When these reports began to emerge in both Europe and the United States, serious efforts were made to protect those who worked with the rays and those who would be exposed to them. These efforts have been successful; today, a career in radiology is as safe as any other career.

ADVANCED EXPERIMENTATION WITH ROENTGEN RAYS

After Roentgen's discovery, most investigators based their experimental priorities on the relationship between x-ray exposure and tissue injury. When the discovery of the roentgen rays was announced throughout the world, several of the investigators who had also been working with cathode rays began to publish literature on their own experiments. It is thought that the first known radiograph

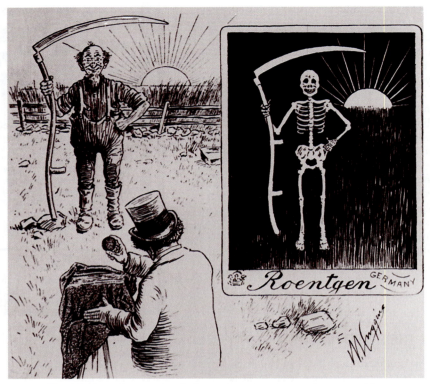

Fig. 4.3 X-ray photography similar to the ones taken at circuses or fairs.

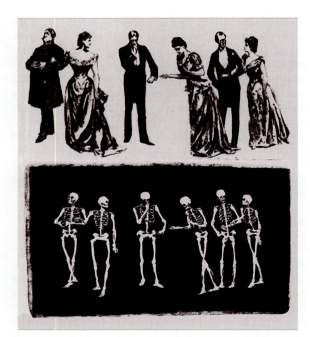

Fig. 4.4 A dangerous party game. (From Glasser O: *Wilhelm Conrad Roentgen and the early history of the roentgen rays,* Springfield, IL, 1933, Charles C. Thomas.)

produced in the United States was made on January 2, 1896, by Michael Idvorsky Pupin, a professor at Columbia University. Pupin's production of the radiograph was thought to have occurred a few days after Roentgen announced his discovery of x-rays.

Soon after the announcement of Roentgen's discovery, Thomas Edison started his experiments with the roentgen rays. His primary concern was working with **fluoroscopy**, a procedure using x-rays to image inner parts of the body in movement and motion. Only after Edison and his staff had performed a large number of experiments did they discover the use of calcium tungstate, a great improvement over barium platinocyanide. Edison promoted the use of calcium tungstate coating in fluoroscopy, with the hope that the vast improvement would increase sales of the fluoroscope. He also became interested in trying to develop a tube in which energy could be transformed into light rather than x-rays. However, he immediately stopped all his research in fluoroscopy, which involved extensive use of radiation, when one of his assistants, Clarence Madison Dally, suffered severe radiation damage as a result of the work.

During the time of Roentgen's work, another field of study evolved. It resulted in the discovery of **radioactivity**, the property of certain elements to emit rays or subatomic particles spontaneously from matter. Three of the most prominent persons credited with this work were Pierre and Marie Curie and Henri Becquerel, who were jointly awarded the Nobel Prize for Physics in 1903. While experimenting with radium on animals, Pierre Curie noticed that the radium killed diseased cells, which was the first suggestion of the medical utility of radioactivity. Marie Curie refined the knowledge of radioactivity and purified the radium metal. In 1911, she received a Nobel Prize for her work in chemistry. She continued to study radioactivity until she developed a severe illness and required a kidney operation. After her health improved, she became acquainted with Albert Einstein and resumed her experiments with radium. However, her efforts were halted because of World War I. Unable to work in her laboratory, she made radiographic equipment for the French military medical service. She developed approximately 20 mobile radiographic units and 200 installations for the army. After training herself as an x-ray technician, she trained French soldiers and gave x-ray classes to American soldiers.

The demand for x-ray equipment and technicians (as they were then called) continued to rise through the years. With the onset of World War II, a shortage of roentgenologists and equipment occurred in the United States because the army was sending technicians and supplies overseas. The US Army established the Army School of Roentgenology at the University of Tennessee at Memphis in 1942. The army continued to train x-ray personnel at John Gaston Hospital in Memphis and trained more than 900 enlisted technicians. These graduates greatly helped relieve the need for qualified technicians.

NUCLEAR RADIOLOGY

Continuous improvements in x-ray equipment brought about several other studies in radiology, including **nuclear radiology**, the branch of radiology using radioactive materials for medical diagnosis and treatment. In 1932, Ernest Lawrence invented the **cyclotron**, a chamber that made it possible to accelerate particles to high speeds for use as projectiles. The cyclotron first made radioisotopes available in large quantities. Enrico Fermi made a significant breakthrough when he induced a successful chain reaction in a uranium pile at the University of Chicago in 1942. The results of this breakthrough were first demonstrated when atomic devices were detonated experimentally in 1945 at White Sands, New Mexico. Shortly thereafter, these devices were introduced as weapons when atomic bombs were dropped on Hiroshima and Nagasaki, Japan. Ironically, from the same basic research that ushered in the age of nuclear arms emerged the highly beneficial medical applications of radioisotopes.

MODERN DIGITAL RADIOGRAPHY

The technical advances in radiology since Roentgen's discovery of x-rays in 1895 have been phenomenal. Today's imaging departments consist of an impressive array of diagnostic capabilities.

For decades, radiographic images were acquired on x-ray film. Numerous companies marketed film and intensifying screens for use in radiographic cassettes. Such film had to be developed in expensive processors using caustic and environmentally unsafe chemicals. Although interest in **digital radiography** existed for many years, it was simply cost prohibitive. As computer technology became mainstream, hardware and software costs dropped, and their capabilities greatly expanded.

Extremely fast **microprocessor speed**, relatively inexpensive **computer memory**, and high-resolution monitors are the technologies that combine to create all-digital radiology departments. X-ray images are acquired using flat plate image receptors whose information is then reconstructed by a computer. The computer manipulates the electronic digital image using **algorithms** to construct the visible image. The resultant image is available on a computer monitor workstation within seconds of the exposure. Upon verification by the radiographer that it is a diagnostic image, it is forwarded to a radiologist for interpretation. Because the image is digital, the radiologist may be within the same department, at home, or anywhere around the world.

Many specialties have emerged in addition to diagnostic radiography, including **computed tomography**, **magnetic resonance imaging**, nuclear medicine, radiation therapy, **diagnostic medical sonography**, and **interventional radiology** (Fig. 4.5). Diagnosing or treating many medical problems would be nearly impossible without this team of radiology modalities.

Continuing education has played an important role in the development of radiology and is essential in keeping abreast of the rapid changes and innovations in the field. Radiology, in its relatively short history, has proved its capabilities and will continue to serve patients in the years to come.

CONCLUSION

It can be seen that the history of radiology is a story of how creative individuals built on the discoveries and inventions of others, adding their own inventive techniques to create the radiologic practices we have today. From the earliest scientists and craftsmen, such as Archimedes and Democritus, to the more current scientists, such as Faraday, Hittorf,

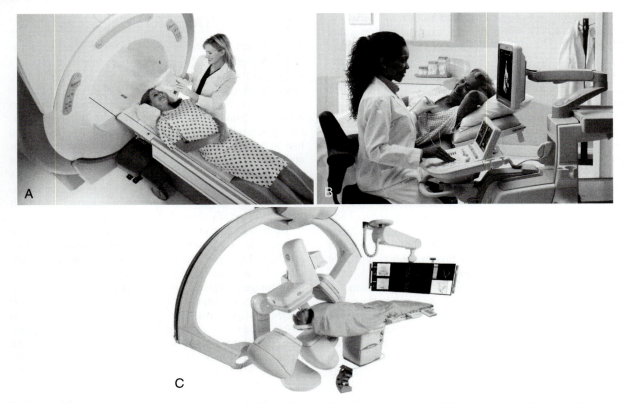

Fig. 4.5 **A,** Magnetic resonance imaging is a medical imaging modality that uses, instead of the x-ray, nonionizing radiofrequency waves, a strong magnetic field, and a computer to produce an image. **B,** Diagnostic medical sonography uses nonionizing sound waves to image internal anatomy. **C,** Interventional radiography allows visualization of the heart and vascular system as well as providing the opportunity to repair or replace diseased vessels. (From Long BW, Rollins JH, et al: *Merrill's atlas of radiographic positioning and procedures*, ed 13, St. Louis, 2016, Elsevier.)

Roentgen, and Edison, we see each one's work building on another's in the development of radiology. In addition, we witness the continuing development of radiologic advances, with improved imaging equipment for more accurate diagnosis and advanced therapeutic units for the treatment of diseases.

QUESTIONS FOR DISCUSSION AND CRITICAL THINKING

1. Construct a timeline illustrating the evolution of radiology.
2. Describe the events surrounding Roentgen's discovery of x-rays.
3. State the role played by Anna Bertha Roentgen.
4. Explain the superfluous use of x-rays in products and entertainment in the years immediately after their discovery and announcement.
5. Describe the role played by computer technology in x-ray imaging.

BIBLIOGRAPHY

Coates JB. *Radiology in World War II.* Washington, DC: Office of the US Surgeon General, Department of the Army; 1966.

Dewing S. *Modern radiology in historical perspective.* Springfield, IL: Charles C Thomas; 1962.

Eisenberg RL. *Radiology: an illustrated history.* St. Louis: Mosby; 1992.

Glasser O: *W.C. Roentgen Dr.*, ed 2, Springfield, IL, 1972, Charles C Thomas.

Glasser O. *Wilhelm Conrad Roentgen and the early history of the roentgen rays.* Springfield, IL: Charles C Thomas; 1933.

Grigg ERN. *The trail of the invisible light.* Springfield, IL: Charles C Thomas; 1965.

Harris EL, et al. *The shadowmakers: a history of radiologic technology.* Albuquerque, NM: American Society of Radiologic Technologists; 1995.

Long B, Rollins J, Smith B. *Merrill's atlas of radiographic positioning and procedures.* ed 14. St. Louis: Elsevier; 2020.

PART II

Practicing the Profession

5

Orientation to Patient Care

OBJECTIVES

On completion of this chapter, you should be able to:
- Describe the defining characteristics of different age groups.
- Discuss how these characteristics will influence your interactions with them.
- Explain the legal implications in dealing with the very young and the very old.
- List the several precautions to take to ensure the patient's safety while he or she is in your care.
- Explain why radiation protection practices are more important for the very young.
- Discuss the legal concerns in reporting patient abuse.
- Prevent injury to the patient during a radiographic examination.
- Protect the patient, yourself, and others from contagious diseases by practicing proper isolation, sterile, and aseptic techniques.
- Reassure and comfort, within the limits of your training, the anxious or fearful patient.
- Use proper body mechanics when moving and transferring patients.
- Discuss the importance of maintaining the existing status of indwelling catheters and other patient attachments.
- Explain what is meant by monitoring vital signs and describe the radiologic technologist's role in this aspect of patient care.
- Discuss the significance of requiring clinical information when radiographic service is requested.
- Explain the importance of recording or charting patient information.

OUTLINE

KEY TERMS

adolescents
antiseptics
body mechanics
cardiac arrest
cardiopulmonary resuscitation
child abuse
contagious diseases
convulsions

disinfectants
elder abuse
fainting
gravity line
infants
isolation unit
law of Bergonie and Tribondeau
legal guardian

pathogens
patient consent
seizures
shock
sphygmomanometer
sterilization
stethoscope
vital signs

KNOWING YOUR PATIENT

In Chapter 2, you learned that all people have the same basic needs, but other needs will arise that are specific to a situation or circumstance. For example, an infant's needs are different from the needs of an adult, and an illness at any age presents different needs. Knowing something about your patients and the characteristics of the different age groups and cultures will help you interact with them while they are in your care. It is true—patient care means CARING for the patient. Patient care is more than passive empathy. Genuine caring is an active endeavor. Your caring involves more than producing a diagnostic quality examination. It involves doing no harm while performing the examination. Using the proper technique is the practical and only acceptable way to prevent harming your patient by unnecessary exposure to radiation.

Hand washing is another practical way to prevent harm to your patient. The importance of hand washing to prevent the spread of infection cannot be overemphasized. These acts of preventing harm apply to all patients. However, specific acts appropriate for the patient are also required. The way you interact with the patient will vary as a result of the differences in patient age, physical condition, gender, and culture.

Age is the most obvious difference in individuals; consequently, age is the first place to begin this discussion.

Infants

Infants are children during the earliest periods of life. They are afraid of two things, falling and loud noises. Safe, gentle handling of the infant while in your care is the first concern. If it is true, as some think, that an individual decides within the first 10 days of life whether he or she likes this world, you would not want your treatment of a newborn to influence this negatively. Although hard evidence for this belief may be difficult to find, gentle handling of a newborn is always in order. You will be interacting with some infants who have to go through a great deal of painful treatments in the first few days of life (Fig. 5.1).

On the first day of an infant's life, he or she can do many things. Importantly, these activities have not been learned; rather, they are reflexes that require no thought and cannot be controlled by will. The grasping reflex can be observed by placing your finger in the palm of the infant's hand. He or she will instantly grasp it tightly with an amazing amount of strength. The infant can stretch, squirm, arch the back, kick, and vigorously wave the arms. These actions are clues that the nerves and muscles are developing normally.

An infant's facial expression is his or her way of communication. Infants need to be held securely and spoken to in a

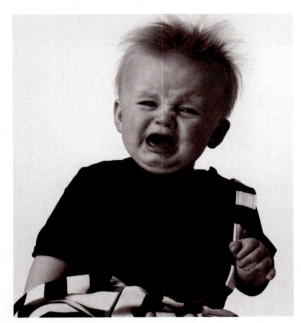

Fig. 5.1 Infants are children during the earliest periods of life. (From Getty Images, Seattle, WA.)

low, soothing voice. A crying, agitated infant will often calm down when wrapped tightly in a blanket and spoken to in a soft, soothing voice. The parent or adult who accompanies the infant can often be a great help in calming the infant and in assisting during the examination.

The first order of safety is preventing physical harm and preventing unwanted exposure or overexposure to radiation. Radiation exposure is more critical to infants than to individuals in any other age group. This is the time to be reminded of the **Law of Bergonie and Tribondeau**, which is based on the sensitivity of cells to ionization radiation. The law states that cells are most sensitive to the effects of ionization radiation when they are rapidly dividing. This is important to remember because the most rapid growth period in an individual's life is during infancy. Cells are dividing very rapidly; thus, infants are most likely to be affected by radiation. When radiographing infants, using radiation protection devices and irradiating only the anatomic part in question are critically important.

Children (1 to 3 Years)

By the time children are 3 years of age, a sense of right and wrong has begun to develop (Fig. 5.2). They have some concept of property and know what belongs to them and what belongs to others. If discipline has been consistent, they will begin to behave in a socially acceptable manner. The behavior may not always be consistent, but children know the

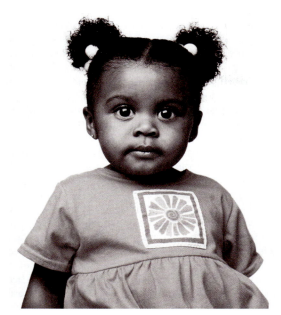

Fig. 5.2 By the time a child is 3 years old, a sense of right and wrong has begun to develop. (From Getty Images, Seattle, WA.)

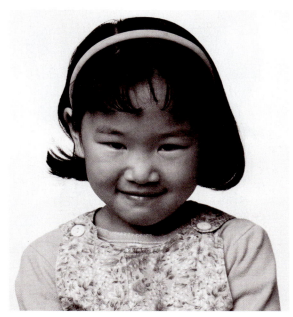

Fig. 5.3 A child develops a sense of self during the wide span of growth years from ages 3 to 12 years. (From Getty Images, Seattle, WA.)

difference between right and wrong. Their reasoning ability may not be developed at this time; that is, they may not know why certain acts are not socially acceptable. In other words, they do not always seem to know what is acceptable and what is not.

They can speak, make sentences, and follow instructions. However, they may choose not to do so, which is often the case. The parent or adult who is accompanying a child will be helpful with this age group as they are with infants. If a child in this age group has had a previously painful experience in a hospital or medical facility, the memory of that experience may evoke a negative response. The parent will be helpful in calming or restraining the child if needed. If time permits, interacting with the child and gaining his or her trust are laudable goals, but the parent will probably be more successful than you.

Children (3 to 12 Years)

During this wide span of growth years, the child's development includes the concept of self (Fig. 5.3). This group has been out in a world that must seem big and confusing. They have new associates; school brings them in contact with others who are not family. Their names become important because this makes them a unit separate from the others. Love and esteem become very important to this age group. The teachers of this group recognize this concept and award

tokens (e.g., gold stars) frequently and liberally to students who accomplish their assigned tasks. This age group has integrated into society and has become socialized as they interact with others in school. Normally, they will have learned to postpone instant gratification for the promise of future gain. This big step indicates that they have developed a concept of time. Communication with this age group should not be a problem. In examinations during which some pain is involved, this age group can normally tolerate some pain knowing that what hurts now will be made well later.

Before leaving the discussion on the interaction with children, it should be mentioned that you will have a special responsibility when examining traumatized or otherwise abused children, especially infants. You may encounter children who have been physically or sexually abused or merely abused because of neglect. In such cases, you should know what is legally required of you. All states have laws regarding who should report abuse, but states differ on these laws. Some states require that anyone who knows of **child abuse** must report it to proper authorities; other states list specific health care professionals as the recipients of reports of child abuse. It is incumbent on the health care provider to know the requirements in his or her state and to recognize injuries that are not consistent with the explanation given as the cause of the injury.

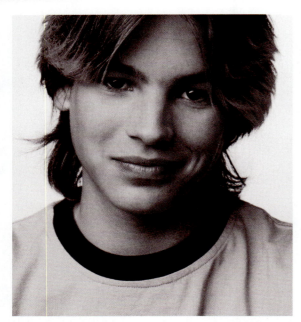

Fig. 5.4 The teenage years are expected to be intense and troubling for both the parents and the adolescent. (From Getty Images, Seattle, WA.)

Adolescents

The teenage years are expected to be intense and troubling for both the parents and the teenager (Fig. 5.4). All training during early childhood has been aimed at making the individual capable of being independent. **Adolescents** want to be independent but do not yet have the skills or maturity to be so; thus, they become frustrated. In addition, a major decision has to be made during this age on what they want to become as adults. This decision can be very difficult for those in this age group. There was a time when a young boy was expected to follow in his father's footsteps and simply continue in the family business or trade. This is not so anymore. Consequently, choosing a career that is attainable can be a real dilemma for many because of the numerous options available to them.

Teenagers want identity and want to be treated as adults. In conversations with them, the adult approach will most likely generate a cooperative response. They may even volunteer information and express an interest in the imaging process or in their scheduled examination. A dominant characteristic of this age group is the close relationships they have with their peer group. In extreme cases, the peer group will have more influence over the teenager than the parents, teachers, or others in authority—sometimes with tragic consequences. Fortunately, these influences diminish in most adolescents as they mature and develop realistic goals and aspirations. As they gain maturity, they will be able to differentiate the possible from the ideal and evaluate and compare different points of view. With this ability, they will encounter and recognize the reality of human failings, which may make them critical of institutions and organizations. Generally, they will come to accept the prevailing expectations of society.

A troubling aspect in treating teenagers—in fact, all children—is figuring out who has the authority to make medical decisions for them. Usually society will seek the permission of the parent or **legal guardian** for all medical treatment for those younger than 18 years of age. However, an underage child may be hurt at school and be brought to the radiology department by a school employee. Sometimes a relative—a grandmother or an older sibling—or even a fellow teenager may be the one who brings the young patient for care. Such situations present a dilemma because these individuals have no legal right to make medical decisions for the child. Instances exist in which the right of the parent to make the medical decision for their child has been questioned. Some parents whose religious beliefs cause them to reject medical help will instead leave the child's fate in the hands of God. There is no clear-cut answer here. This medical dilemma is outside the scope of this text.

Young Adults (21 to 45 Years)

A teenager, impatient to become independent, is now an adult with responsibilities and obligations not merely for his or her own welfare but also, in most individuals, for the welfare of others (Fig. 5.5). Most have selected a partner because they have a critical need for intimacy, have started a family, have settled into a career or job, and have established a place in the community. Young adulthood is a period of productive and creative effort. However, it is also a time when problems arise as the new role of responsibility for taking care of family, financially and in other ways, becomes demanding and stressful.

In the event of a life-threatening disease, young adult patients may appear to be overly concerned about their health. Their anxiety is understandable and should be expected. A life-threatening illness at this untimely age can be devastating. They are not only concerned about their own welfare, but they may also have dependents whose lives will be drastically altered without their support.

You will be able to interact with this adult group because, generally, they are able to understand and follow instructions. Being a good listener is appropriate with this age group.

Middle Age (45 to 65 Years)

Those in this age group will have settled into sharing their lives with others (Fig. 5.6). They have developed a pattern of

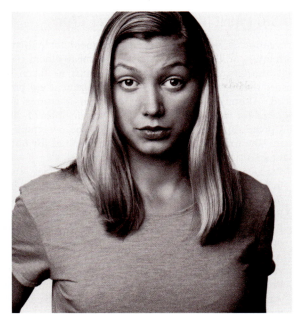

Fig. 5.5 Teenagers, impatient to become independent, are now adults with obligations and the responsibility for not only their own welfare but also, in many individuals, for the welfare of others. (From Getty Images, Seattle, WA.)

activity with their families and communities. Their children are becoming independent, the "empty nest syndrome" may cause them to seek a greater role in civic and community affairs, and they may travel or seek other diversions apart from family. They have a well-defined value system and associate with others with similar values. Their concerns may be in maintaining their independence and preparing for the years after retirement. Your interaction with this group will be similar to that in the previous age group.

Senior Citizens (65 Years and Older)

This country and nations all around the world are experiencing a population growth of people over 50 years of age (Fig. 5.7). The fastest growing segment of this country's population today is people older than 85 years of age. Of this segment of the population, 70% are women. Approximately 100 years ago, women died younger than men, many in childbirth. The life expectancy was only 47 years. Today, life expectancy is over 79 years.

The majority of this group will suffer from such diseases as osteoporosis, diabetes, arthritis, Alzheimer disease, cancer, and heart and vascular diseases. Despite this litany of diseases affecting the aging population, many continue to be active, productive citizens. Older people, some advanced in years, continue working. Many are volunteers, performing

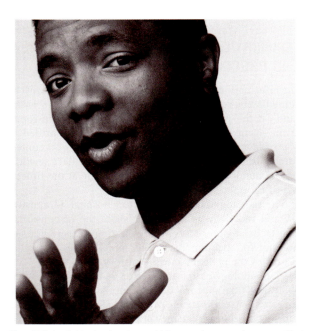

Fig. 5.6 Individuals in the middle-aged group have settled into sharing their lives with others. (From Getty Images, Seattle, WA.)

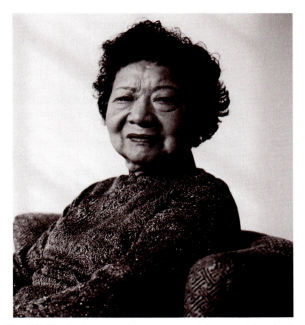

Fig. 5.7 The fastest growing segment of the population in the United States today is made up of people older than 85 years of age. (From Getty Images, Seattle, WA.)

useful tasks; some take enrichment courses and even start new careers.

These patients need to be treated as any other adult—with dignity and respect. They may move more slowly and may require support. Many have difficulty hearing and seeing, and communicating with these patients may be difficult. Obviously, you will have patients in this age group who are terminally ill. Some will not be able to respond to your instructions. They need to be handled gently, taking care to make them as comfortable as the examination permits. It may be necessary to call for assistance in examining patients who are unable to understand or respond to instructions. Dealing with death and dying patients is beyond the scope of this text, but it is not beyond the scope of your curriculum in radiography. Understanding the process—the emotional, physical, and personal aspects of death—is an essential component of your education.

The increased life expectancy of people today has placed the responsibility of caring for them on others. For some individuals, this added responsibility has been stressful and has resulted in **elder abuse**, often by mere neglect. Elder abuse is becoming more common, and the abuse may be physical, financial, or psychologic. As with child abuse, states differ when it comes to the laws regarding elder abuse. What is different in elder abuse is that the patient must sign a **patient consent** form to have the abuse legally reported.

Diverse Conditions and Populations

Most of the discussions in the preceding topics have been about the average or the usual patient. However, you will encounter patients who may exhibit problems beyond the average and patients who merely require special treatment. For example, patients of a different culture who speak a different language may require special attention in your interaction with them. Your duty in situations such as these is to respect the patient's beliefs. If language is a problem, calling for assistance in communicating to the patient may be necessary to ensure that a diagnostic examination can be performed.

Other patients who will present different problems are those who abuse alcohol or drugs, who have a communicable disease, and those who have suffered trauma. In addition, you will interact with patients undergoing treatment with catheters, tubes, orthopedic equipment, or other medical devices attached. These conditions and situations require knowledge and skill and, in some cases, innovation. One answer will not fit all. Each case presents its own unique challenge, but every patient requires the radiographer to act in a caring manner. Remember, most patients are dealing with pain, anxiety, and fear, and your interactions with them must always be respectful, courteous, and professional.

BASIC PRINCIPLES OF PATIENT CARE

Prevention is always better than treatment for patients with injury or illness, but no one is immune to illness, natural disasters, or human error. Care must be taken to ensure that good patient care and management are provided. Although we know that different measures are required for varying circumstances, the principles of care and protection are constant and cannot be overemphasized. The following requirements are required for optimal patient care:

1. Practice high-quality radiographic techniques that include radiation safety in a manner that will minimize further injury or complications.
2. Prevent the spread of disease and injury to others.
3. Prevent hazardous or crippling complications of injuries or illnesses.
4. Alleviate suffering by comforting the patient and preventing emotional complications.
5. Provide the service as economically and in as timely a way as possible while maintaining consistent diagnostic quality.

To ensure that these five requirements are met, certain policies and procedures are necessary. These may be written in detail in the hospital or department policy manual and will serve as the basis for performing certain patient care functions.

VERIFICATION OF PATIENT IDENTIFICATION AND PROCEDURES REQUESTED

The information on the examination request form must be immediately verified or matched to the patient's wristband on the patient's arrival to the radiographic room. In the event that the patient has not been identified or is unable to give identification, an emergency control number should be assigned with hospital chart verification so that a cross-reference can be made at the time of identification.

The radiology physician director, hospital administrator, and radiology administrator share the responsibility for establishing procedures for requesting radiographic service and for maintaining radiographic images and other records of the patient's medical history.

The radiology physician director maintains the responsibility and final approval of the examination requested and can cancel or terminate the procedure at any point. Clinical information about pregnancy or possible pregnancy or precautions to be observed because of special conditions such as deafness, blindness, diabetes, heart problems, and allergies are required in most departments.

Patient Transfer

Often a medical emergency occurs when a patient is transported to or from the radiographic suite or in the radiographic area. Therefore, all students or radiology staff involved in patient care must be qualified in **cardiopulmonary resuscitation** (CPR), which is the restoration of function of the heart and lungs after apparent death. Transport equipment such as wheelchairs, stretchers, and beds should be kept in proper working order. Ancillary equipment such as step stools and intravenous stands must also be maintained, and preventive maintenance safety checks should be conducted often. On arrival at the patient area, an assessment of the patient's condition and wristband identification should be made. The ability of the patient to be ambulatory, the patient's injury, and the auxiliary equipment necessary for the patient's condition must be observed, as well as any further precautions noted on the requisition.

Patients must be informed as to where they are to be transported, and assistance must be given when necessary to ensure safe and comfortable transport. The responsible unit personnel should be advised of the patient's destination. Care should be taken to ensure safety to both the patient and the employee. If the transporter needs assistance, the patient should not be moved until such time that sufficient trained staff is available.

Proper **body mechanics** (i.e., the action of muscles in producing motion or posture) can best be practiced by employees who have been trained in such techniques. Although a detailed discussion is not appropriate in this text, a few salient points may be helpful. The most important point to keep in mind is that, at all times, human action is influenced by gravity. The center of gravity in a standing human being is at the center of the pelvis. Equilibrium or balance is maintained when the **gravity line** passes through the base support; the gravity line is an imaginary vertical line that passes through the center of gravity. Stability of a body is increased by broadening the base support. Therefore, balance is maintained more easily with the feet spread apart than when they are positioned close together. When lifting or moving a patient, you should use this advantage and spread your feet slightly to maintain your balance and stability. Lowering the center of gravity also increases stability. The amount of muscular effort required to maintain stability is directly related to the height of the center of gravity and to the breadth of the base support. Therefore, to conserve energy and to reduce the strain on your muscles when lifting or moving patients, lower your body's center of gravity and broaden your base of support. When lifting an object from the floor, you should bend your knees because this serves as a shock absorber; do not bend from your waist. When lifting a patient, spread your feet slightly to increase your base support and hold the patient close to your body so that the center of gravity is balanced over both of your feet. Protect your spine by using your arm and leg muscles (Fig. 5.8).

The following list presents some general principles to follow when moving or lifting patients:

1. Place your body in the correct position before moving or lifting.
2. Place your feet far enough apart to maintain proper balance and to provide a basis of support.
3. Hold the patient as close as possible to your body to eliminate all unnecessary strain by centralizing the total weight within your grasp.
4. Stoop to the working level, and keep your back straight.
5. Slide rather than lift whenever possible.
6. When a patient is too heavy for you to move alone, get help.
7. When two or more people are moving or lifting, give a signal, and move or lift in unison.

The patient should be encouraged to help with the move if he or she is able. Because patients will most likely be slow in their response to your instructions, patience may be required. Allowing patients to help themselves preserves their sense of independence and control over illness.

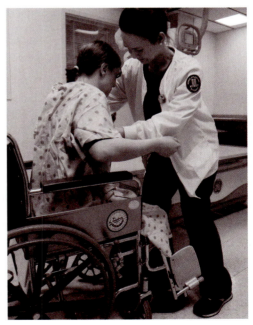

Fig. 5.8 Spreading the feet slightly and holding the patient close to your body to ensure that the center of gravity is balanced over both feet increases stability and protects the back muscles. (Courtesy of Courtney Hensley and Jessica Gordan, Methodist University Hospital; Joseph Martin, photographer.)

The transporter and all radiology staff in patient care should be thoroughly comfortable with the use, identification, and operation of equipment and attachments such as catheters, oxygen masks, drainage tubes, and electrocardiogram (ECG) electrodes. Proper attention must be given to ensure that tubes and catheters remain intact and free of contamination. The hospital department of radiology manual may contain policies and procedures for the care of patients who have equipment attached. The responsibility of the radiologic technologists in monitoring and adjusting the equipment should be stated in the radiology policy and procedures manual. Large departments may employ a technologist with advanced training to adjust and check drainage tubes and other equipment that is attached to the patient. However, regardless of who is assigned the responsibility, you should know some of the most commonly encountered auxiliary equipment and how to care for the patient to whom it is attached; the general rule is to maintain the unit in its present state and to prevent contamination. Fainting, shock, seizures, cardiac arrest, convulsions, loss of consciousness, and bleeding are conditions that must be managed if and when they occur. (**Fainting** is a sudden fall in blood pressure with the loss of consciousness. **Shock** is the profound depression of the vital functions with reduced blood volume and pressure, usually caused by severe injuries. **Seizures** are attacks such as convulsions or the sudden onset of a disease. **Cardiac arrest** is a state of complete cessation of the heart's action. **Convulsions** are violent, involuntary muscular contractions or spasms.)

All radiology personnel and students in any patient care area should have the ability to monitor **vital signs**, which include blood pressure, temperature, pulse, and respiration. They should also be able to use a **stethoscope** (i.e., an instrument used to hear respiratory and cardiac sounds), thermometer, and **sphygmomanometer** (i.e., an instrument that measures blood pressure). Recording vital signs information on the hospital chart, radiology requisition, or incident report form is provided in accordance with imaging department policy. Requesting information about these matters as the need for it arises is partially the responsibility of the student. Changes from the routine radiographic procedures must be considered. For example, a patient with myelomeningocele or osteogenesis imperfecta must be handled with extreme care. When working with a patient with a colostomy or ileostomy, the special guidelines involved in removing and replacing receptor bags must be followed. The intravenous infusion check is an important consideration of care that is needed in the radiology department. Emergency medications and equipment carts must be available and properly maintained at all times in the radiology department.

Isolation Techniques

Special care must be taken to prevent patients from acquiring a hospital-related infection. These are known as health care-acquired infections and are the cause of thousands of deaths every year. Equipment should be wiped with disinfectant solution after each radiographic examination (Fig. 5.9).

Significant research was conducted by Dr. Mary Loritsch of Virginia Western Community College and Sonya Lawson of Virginia Commonwealth University to determine the presence of **pathogens** on radiography equipment and accessories. It was found that pathogens can live and even colonize on radiographic equipment. This research is significant because it points out the importance of cleanliness in the operation of a radiology department. Patients visiting the radiology department should not risk getting another infection in addition to the condition that they already have (Lawson, Sauer, and Loritsch, 2002).

Preventing the spread of diseases is an important consideration in all hospitals and in any other patient care facilities. These are called standard precautions, the most important of which is hand washing before and after caring for each patient. The Centers for Disease Control and Prevention publishes guidelines for isolation precautions in hospitals specifically for patients with communicable diseases. Hospital procedure manuals include these guidelines and make them a part of orientation for new employees and radiography students.

You may be called on to perform an examination in an **isolation unit**; therefore, you should be acquainted with the procedures for entering and leaving such an area. When

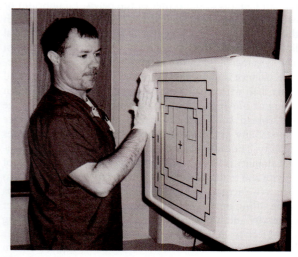

Fig. 5.9 Cleaning radiographic equipment. (Courtesy of John Sullivan, Methodist University Hospital.)

performing radiographic examinations in an isolation unit, special clothing may be required, which usually consist of a gown, cap, mask, and gloves. The purposes of an isolation unit are to confine the disease to the patient, to protect the people working with the patient, and to protect other patients. It may also be used to protect the patient from microorganisms carried by people entering the unit. All equipment and accessories must be made readily available, but they must not come in contact with the patient until the immediate time of use. Cassettes should be placed in a pillowcase during the examination. The case housing of the radiographic equipment should be wiped with disinfectant solution before leaving the unit. **Disinfectants** are substances that are used to destroy pathogens (i.e., viruses, microorganisms, or other substances causing disease) or to render them inert. **Antiseptics** are substances that prevent or retard the growth of microorganisms; alcohol is a commonly used antiseptic in hospitals.

Department isolation techniques require very strict procedures if the disease is contagious. **Contagious diseases** such as chickenpox, tuberculosis, herpes zoster, measles, and mumps may be contracted by droplet or airborne routes. Other diseases may be contracted by direct or indirect contact only and thus require a different isolation technique. Typical of these are bacterial and viral infections such as *Salmonella* spp. and *Escherichia coli* and other diseases that affect the bowel with resultant infected feces. Strict isolation techniques are used for patients with diphtheria, eczema vaccinatum, draining lesions, German measles, and smallpox. Protective isolation is used to protect a susceptible patient from becoming infected, as in the case of patients with burns or leukemia. Infants in critical care nurseries and patients with open lesions are also candidates for the isolation unit.

For the practice of aseptic techniques, the most important precaution is hand washing; often, unfortunately, hand washing is the most neglected practice.

Patients with wounds or those in respiratory isolation can be brought into the department of radiology. However, few other patients should be present, and these patients must be kept separate, examined quickly, and promptly returned to their units. After the examination, the radiographic room, table, and equipment used must be promptly disinfected as protocol specifies. These practices should also be exercised for the patient in protective isolation, with the additional requirement that the radiology staff wear face masks when in the presence of the patient.

Sterile or Aseptic Techniques

The surgical department's aseptic technique is an inherent practice within that unit, and the radiologic technologist

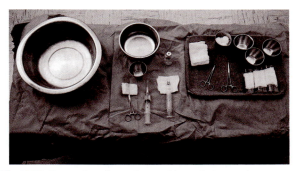

Fig. 5.10 Opened sterile package with sterile items that are typically used in special radiographic procedures.

must exercise constant watchfulness to avoid contaminating sterile objects and the reserved space on the surgical side of the table (Fig. 5.10).

Sterilization implies the complete removal or destruction of microorganisms. It is beyond the scope of this text to describe fully the techniques for providing a sterile field for practicing aseptic techniques. The following items are based on the major principles of the techniques and are offered as a guide:

1. An article is either sterile or unsterile; there is no in between. If any doubt exists, you must consider the article to be unsterile.
2. Sterile articles must be kept covered until ready for use.
3. Only the outside of the wrapper or cover is touched when opening a sterile package or container.
4. A sterile article is handled with a sterile instrument or sterile gloves.
5. After an article is removed from a sterile container, it is not to be returned to that container.
6. When removing an article from a sterile container, use the forceps provided. Only that part of the container and the part of the forceps that is covered by disinfecting solution are considered sterile. Always hold the tip of the forceps downward. Remove the cover of the container. Hold the cover in one hand. Remove the article with the forceps in the other hand. Replace the cover. If you must lay down the cover, turn it upside down on a flat surface.
7. When a container becomes contaminated, dispose of it at once. If you cannot do it immediately, turn the cover to show it is contaminated.
8. Avoid reaching over a sterile field.
9. Edges of sterile towels are considered contaminated after contact with an unsterile surface.
10. Keep instrument handles out of sterile fields.

11. Pour sterile solutions so that no contact between the bottle and the sides of the container occurs.

Aseptic techniques and special patient considerations must be a part of the department's overall policy routine for preparing syringes; patient prepping; disposal of needles, catheters, and tubes; and cleanup. When medication is administered, great care must be taken. The proper drug, the prescribed amount, how it is to be administered, that is, whether intravenously or via another route, and the time the medication is given are items requiring special attention. Charting or recording information about the patient's condition and your role in the patient's examination is an important parts of patient care, especially so in the case of an accident in which the outcome may be in question. The team concept in isolation or special patient consideration must be exercised at all times.

CONCLUSION

In your course of study to become a radiographer, you will learn specific ways to interact with several types of patients seeking radiologic service. Generally, the most difficult patients will be the very young and the very old. These are the patients who need the most gentle care. As a professional, you will be able to use judgment and logic in the performance of your duties, knowing that your patient is depending on you for a diagnostic examination.

The underlying objective for discussing patient care and management is to provide safety for the patient and for those who work with patients in radiology. Quality radiographic techniques must include patient-handling tasks that are necessary to prevent injury, the spread of disease, and other hazardous complications.

QUESTIONS FOR DISCUSSION AND CRITICAL THINKING

1. Compare and contrast the characteristics associated with each age group and how they impact patient care.
2. Discuss the importance of accurate patient identification.
3. Explain the importance of proper body mechanics to both patient and radiographer.
4. Explain why the radiographer must be knowledgeable of all types of biomedical equipment and patient conditions.
5. Discuss the critical importance of infection control.
6. Relate hand washing to infection control.

BIBLIOGRAPHY

Chatman J, et al. *Behavior and health care: a humanistic and helping process.* St. Louis: Mosby; 1975.

de Cecco J, et al. *The psychology of learning and instruction: educational psychology*, ed 2. Englewood Cliffs, NJ: Prentice-Hall; 1974.

Ehrlich RA, McCloskey ED, Daly JA. *Patient care in radiography*, ed 7. St. Louis: Mosby; 2008.

Kushma D. *The commercial appeal the graying of the globe.* *Memphis Daily News*, April 5, 2002.

Lawson SR, Sauer R, Loritsch MB. Bacterial survival on radiographic cassettes. *Radiol Technol.* 2002; 73(6):507–510.

Leafer C. Getting it right, writing it down, the technologist's role in charting. *Radiol Today.* 2004; 5(19):14.

Long B, Rollins J, Smith B. *Merrill's atlas of radiographic positioning and procedures.* ed 14. Elsevier: St. Louis; 2020.

Radiology Specialist Program (JP90350), Boulder, CO, 1958, School of Aviation Medicine, USAF Air University.

Smith M. Aging is just another word for living. *Vital Speeches of the Day* LXIX. 2003;(7):212–215.

Snopek AM. *Fundamentals of special radiographic procedures.* ed 4. Saunders; 2006.

Spieler G. New environment, challenges and triumphs moving from pediatrics and geriatrics. *ASRT Scanner.* 2006; 38(12):14–15.

Wilson B. *Ethics and basic law for medical imaging professionals.* Philadelphia: FA Davis; 1997.

6

Providing Quality Patient Service

OBJECTIVES

On completion of this chapter, you should be able to:
- Explain the importance of having a thorough understanding of the technical aspects of radiologic technology.
- Name the sources of information that most patients use when choosing a hospital.
- List the inside and outside customers served by the health care facility.
- Discuss the variety of diversity among patients.

- Describe quality care from the patient's perspective.
- List high-tech and high-touch aspects of health care.
- Explain what is meant by a *moment of truth.*
- Outline a customer service cycle for a radiologic examination.
- List ways to enhance telephone conversations.
- Define *empathy.*
- Be able to use the conflict resolution model in customer service and in high-stress situations.

OUTLINE

KEY TERMS

conflict resolution
customer service cycle
diversity
effective listening

empathy
events
incidents
inside customers

moments of truth
outside customers

Radiography is first and foremost a people-oriented business. It carries with it special opportunities. Patients have entrusted their health to us, and they need to believe they are in the best of hands. Consequently, it is up to you, as a new health care professional, to dedicate yourself to providing the highest quality of care and service to your patients.

OVERVIEW: THE HEALTH CARE SERVICE ENVIRONMENT

One of the most important facets of your practice is the realization that you are part of a service industry. Patients and their families are, in fact, customers. Many health care professionals are uncomfortable using the term *customer* for those served in the hospital; therefore, the term *patient* is used in this book when appropriate. However, keep in mind that a customer is someone to whom we provide a product or service, and this definition describes a patient perfectly. Although our product is quite different from that of other service businesses, we are, nevertheless, judged by many of the same criteria. Total patient care must be a balance of human caring and concern, technical expertise, and high-quality customer service. Caring and quality service are not mutually exclusive; in fact, only when these aspects of care are combined in the health care setting are we able to satisfy the needs of our patients and provide the quality they have come to expect. Any one of these traits, on its own, does not provide total patient care.

Keep in mind that patients and the services we offer them should never be thought of in exactly the same vein as fast-food restaurants, department stores, and hotels. If quality service is expected and delivered in those service settings, then we, as health care professionals, can certainly provide similar levels of service for our patients and practices, which are so much more important.

The Joint Commission (TJC) stipulates that patient and family complaint systems must be in place and available for use as part of a continuous quality improvement program. Furthermore, TJC specifies that such complaint systems allow grievances relating to the quality of care to be addressed. In addition, the Centers for Medicare & Medicaid Services (CMS) bases part of its payment on patient satisfaction scores calculated from the surveys they perform.

Service systems, strategies, and people form the basis for marketing and service delivery in today's successful health care organizations. Thus, hospitals are focused on delivering the quality of service that an increasingly demanding public expects.

A good understanding of the health care delivery system is vital to student radiographers because this delivery system is the context in which all patient care takes place. You will be a part of this system from the beginning of school and throughout your career. In your role as a student and later as an employee, you must be able to function within the socioeconomic boundaries of health care delivery. A strong grasp of these concepts is vital to being a productive member of the health care team. Most important, however, are the interactions you will have with your patients.

THE PATIENT'S PERSPECTIVE

Who are our patients? From where do our patients come? What do our patients think, and what do they expect? How do we begin to understand them and their specific needs? For health care professionals, these questions are not easily answered. However, a good place to start is with the understanding that although many differences exist among people of all backgrounds, we are all more alike than different.

Humans respond positively to kindness and respect. People want to feel safe and secure, especially in an unfamiliar environment. They want to be comfortable. Patients want to be free of pain and discomfort. Privacy is important, as is the comfort of the family. People who become our patients want their individual beliefs, wants, and needs accommodated as much as possible.

Diversity among individuals is infinite; the gene pool of over 8 billion people produces infinite combinations. Each person is unique. Every human being is then influenced not only by a specific culture but by life experiences. Some studies focus on cultural diversity alone, but such an approach will severely limit your understanding of your patients. Regardless of an individual's cultural background, life will add things such as age, illness, injury, and socioeconomics, to name only a few. Gender, family tradition, sexual preference, and religious beliefs are all part of each patient's background.

As you begin working with patients in clinical education, you will discover that every patient brings unique experiences and a view of life that you have not yet experienced. Patients will also teach you the folly of stereotypes; no matter the background of the patient, broad judgments must never be made to fit preconceived notions.

Cultural diversity itself is difficult to define. In the United States, the predominant cultures may be a mix of influences from Europe, Hispanic nations, the continent of Africa, the lands of Asia and the Middle East, and Native American tribes. Some patients may be first-generation immigrants, who are attempting to assimilate into a new culture while still heavily influenced by their culture of origin. Others may be several generations removed from their family's land of origin but still influenced by those beliefs or observe certain traditions or rites. Although bearing physical resemblance to their ancestors, still others may have broken ties with their family's past. As a health care professional, you can never be sure of your patients' backgrounds, regardless of physical appearances. You will need to be comfortable working with a diverse population.

To make a discussion of diversity relevant, consider the ways in which you add to diversity. Think about (better yet, write a page about) your own family heritage; your age; attitudes; socioeconomic status; gender; core religious, moral, and ethical values; preferences in life; sense of humor; diseases or injuries that influence how you live your daily life; privacy or openness; land of origin; and so on. Consider your hopes and dreams, successes and disappointments, victories and failures. Now, picture yourself as a patient. Finally, consider all the variations on your beliefs that might come from over 8 billion human beings.

Your studies in health care include further discussion of diversity, including Chapter 5 of this text. However, some basic considerations should be added to your radiography practice to help you shape your approach to those of diverse backgrounds. Incorporating the key points in Box 6.1 into your practice can enhance interaction and communication with patients. As you read them, keep in mind that references to cultures and limited English-speaking individuals can also refer to older adults, very young patients, seriously impaired patients, and others. Consider that these suggestions may be used in a multitude of situations, with a wide variety of patients who may not necessarily be from another country or culture.

BOX 6.1   Key Points for Diverse Patient Interactions

Tips for Successful Caregiver and Patient Interaction Across Cultures

1. Don't treat the patient in the same manner you would want to be treated.
2. Begin by being more formal with patients who were born in another culture.
3. Don't be *put off* if the patient fails to *look you in the eye* or to ask questions about the treatment.
4. Don't make *any* assumptions regarding the patient's concepts about the ways to maintain health, the causes of illness, or the means to prevent or cure illness.

Tips for Communicating Directly with Limited English-Speaking Patients

1. Speak slowly, not loudly.
2. Face the patient and make extensive use of gestures, pictures, and facial expressions. Watch the patient's face, eyes, and body language carefully.
3. Avoid difficult and uncommon words and idiomatic expressions.
4. Don't "muddy the waters" with unnecessary words or information.
5. Organize what you say for easy access.
6. Rephrase and summarize often.
7. Don't ask questions that can be answered by yes or no.

From Salimbene S: *What language does your patient hurt in?* ed 1, St. Paul, 2000, Paradigm.

You may be surprised by the suggestion to not treat the patient in the same manner as you would want to be treated. The individuality of each person from the perspective of differing ages, cultures, and backgrounds must remain foremost in your mind. Certainly, a calm and gentle demeanor is universally appropriate, but figures of speech, the use of touch, or an overall approach you might consider normal or even desirable may be offensive to someone else. Asking an older patient if she wishes to hang out in the waiting room may be misinterpreted. Few health care professionals touch the patient as much as a radiographer. You may appreciate a gentle touch of encouragement, but touch must be carefully approached, whether positioning for a procedure or providing encouragement with a hand on the patient's shoulder. Your preferences may not be the same as those of the patients you serve. The ongoing study of diversity of all kinds will greatly assist you with patient interactions. Age and culture greatly influence how a patient interprets your words and actions. Choose them carefully.

Each patient is someone's daughter or son and perhaps someone's mother or father, grandmother or grandfather, brother or sister. Each is unique, with basic wants and needs quite possibly similar to your own, but each patient may wish to be approached in a special way. You must care for each as a valued member of humanity.

Patients as Informed Consumers

Service as expected by the patient and delivered by the caregiver is the prime factor in patient satisfaction. We can attempt to focus on how to provide our services only by knowing what the public perceives about health care delivery.

Consumer organizations regularly interview patients about current issues in health care delivery. Their responses are part of major surveys of the changing health care climate. The information in these surveys is not simply a part of a lesson to be learned; it should be totally integrated into your radiography practice as a member of the health care team. In a field that is as rich in modern technology as is diagnostic imaging and therapy, maintaining a balance between this high technology and the high-touch care that only you can provide is imperative.

Patients are increasingly indicating quality of patient care as crucial in their choice of health care providers. Surveys indicate a strong reliance on word-of-mouth advertising and peer recommendation when selecting physicians and hospitals. However, information gathered from researching the internet is the most common source of health care information. Furthermore, staff courtesy is identified as a very important factor in patients' initial choice of a hospital and their reasons for returning to that hospital. Patients prefer hospitals and clinics that are close to their home. Hence, we see the proliferation of prompt care and walk-in clinics. Health care advertising has been shown to be effective in educating patients about services offered.

The balance between high-tech and high-touch care can be a primary reason for patient satisfaction. It is a focal point for an American public who is better informed and more assertive than at any other time in the history of health care delivery. Your success as a radiographer will be determined by how far you can exceed your patients' expectations.

INSIDE AND OUTSIDE CUSTOMERS

The marketing of health care targets both outside customers and inside customers. Outside customers are those people from outside the hospital such as patients, their families, physicians, and others within the community. Inside customers are members of other departments (e.g., nursing units, emergency department), coworkers, and radiologists.

When we realize that we serve inside customers, the work environment becomes more cooperative. We are as responsible for providing high-quality service to each other as we are for providing it to the patient. All departments are striving to heal those who come to them; we must work together with support and cooperation.

Everyone in the community is an outside customer. We focus on the patients and their families as our primary outside customers; they are the ones who come to us and place their confidence in our care. The physicians who practice at our facility are important outside customers as well. They admit their patients because of our expertise. These physicians also deserve the best of our service.

Many others from the outside come to our facility on a regular basis. They may be suppliers, delivery personnel, clergy, or sales and service specialists. Although they may not be customers, as such, remember that they spread our reputation by word of mouth and should be regarded as important links to the community.

Understanding that we serve both inside and outside customers by providing the care and service they expect and deserve enhances our self-image as radiographers and emphasizes the importance of the role we play within the organization.

BENEFITS OF HIGH-QUALITY SERVICE

Delivering high-quality customer service benefits everyone. Radiographers, the inside and outside customers, and the employer all gain when patient care takes place within the context of a value-added service. Radiographers can

add value by making each interaction special for the person served. Smiles, appropriate touch, using the person's name, explaining the examination, and other examples described in this chapter are all ways of adding value. However, radiographers must be aware that they cannot give away what they do not have; their ability to deliver high-quality care is directly related to self-image, self-esteem, self-confidence, and their values relating to life and the workplace.

MOMENTS OF TRUTH IN RADIOLOGY

High-touch radiography may occur during each moment of an interaction between the patient and the radiographer who is delivering the service. These moments of truth can be considered points at which patients form perceptions about the quality of service being given and, in this case, the quality of care. Such moments of truth begin with observations that the patient makes and conclude with inferences being made about the care and service being provided.

Moments of truth can occur in every conceivable circumstance. They may relate to the physical appearance of the work area, the appearance of the radiographer, and the professional behavior of everyone involved.

You must first realize that quality must be the hallmark of practicing radiography. Understanding that the patient's experiences are a series of moments of truth sets the stage for clinical excellence.

SERVICE CYCLES IN RADIOLOGY

The achievement of patient satisfaction is not something that can be left to chance. By viewing the patient's experiences as cycles, we can examine the events and incidents that make up those cycles. Each customer service cycle is part of the patient's total experience while at the facility or when interacting over the telephone. Divided into its component parts, the radiographer can manage the cycle like acts in a play to ensure that quality service is delivered to each patient. For example, a patient may be scheduled for an outpatient upper gastrointestinal (GI) series (Box 6.2).

BOX 6.2   Service Cycle—Outpatient Upper Gastrointestinal Series

Events
Scheduling the appointment
Arriving at the hospital
Being registered
Having the examination performed
Being released

Having the examination performed and being released are the primary events involving the radiographer; they are made up of incidents (Box 6.3) that are managed by the radiographer.

The key to value-added service is making the patient's experience as pleasant as possible at each step along the way and making it superior to what would be received anywhere else; the challenge is to perform each incident as if you were the best radiographer in the world. As you learn radiographic positioning and procedures, keep in mind that they are but combinations of a series of experiences that can each be enhanced for the patient. Remember that you want to perform each step in the most professional way possible. You want to convey to the patient that you are a competent and reliable professional in whom trust can be placed. Each incident in the list can be enhanced with value-added service as described in the suggestions that follow. Remember, no single best way exists to add value. As a radiographer, you may wish to have many different ways of handling each situation to take into account different patients and examinations and to avoid sounding like a recording.

Each incident may be managed as follows:

1. The use of a patient's name and, if appropriate, his or her title, conveys respect. Adults (those older than approximately 18 to 21 years of age) should not be greeted by their first names. Greeting people with a smile and a handshake is the accepted business salutation in the US culture. It is highly appropriate in health care. EXAMPLE: "Good morning, Mrs. Davidson. My name is Amy Kim. I am the radiographer who will be performing your x-ray examination today".

   When caring for pediatric patients, the use of their first name may ease their anxiety, as well as that of their parents. EXAMPLE: "Good afternoon, Mrs. Anderson. How is Mariah doing today?" or "Hi, Freddy. How are you today?" or "Madi, can I take your picture today?"

2. Instructing the patient on how to dress for the examination makes the patient feel more at ease. Many radiographic examinations require that the patient change into a hospital gown; this can be very uncomfortable for many people. EXAMPLE (on the way to and at the dressing room): "Mrs. Makenna, your x-ray examination requires that you wear a gown with no buttons or snaps that could show up on the x-ray image. You may change into one here in the women's dressing room. Please remove your clothing from the waist up. A locker is provided for your clothing. Be sure to keep your valuables and the key with you. Please have a seat here when you have changed. I will be back as soon as you are ready."

3. Taking the patient to the radiographic examination room may take seconds if it is nearby or minutes if it is located elsewhere in the imaging department. This time may be filled by asking the patient about the registration process, parking, or ease of finding the department. These questions indicate your desire to see that the moments of truth that the patient has already experienced at your institution have been positive. Even if you are not in a position to change an event that the patient has already experienced, asking shows that you care about how events have been handled. This interest offers the patient the opportunity to vent frustration over a mishandled event or to reinforce an already positive experience. In either case, the patient will be more cooperative for you as you perform the examination. EXAMPLE: "Did you have any problems finding a place to park this morning?" (The patient's response indicates that there was a problem.) "I'm sorry to hear that, Mrs. Davidson. I'm sure that was quite annoying. I will let the appropriate department know. They are really trying to improve the situation. When we are finished, I'll give you instructions on how to get back to the parking lot."

4. Taking the patient's history greatly assists the radiologist in interpreting the radiographs. It is yet another opportunity to interact professionally with the patient and to provide value-added service. EXAMPLE: "May I ask why you are having a stomach x-ray examination, Mrs. Davidson? Have you had any difficulty swallowing, a chronic stomach ache, or heartburn? I will share this information with our radiologist so that it may be considered when your images are read."

5. Your careful explanation of the examination gains the patient's cooperation and builds trust in you as a professional. Speaking to the patient during the examination makes the experience more pleasant and helps the patient remain at ease. EXAMPLE: The steps in an upper GI series may be described at this point; you can then add the following: "Do you have any questions about the procedure, Mrs. Davidson? I will be here with you throughout the examination."

6. Your enthusiasm about physicians, other departments, or coworkers conveys that the patient is in good hands. The introduction of the radiologist provides such an opportunity. EXAMPLE (before the radiologist enters the room): "Dr. Kailin Alexander, an excellent radiologist, will be performing the first part of your examination today." (When the radiologist enters the room) "Mrs. Davidson, I would like you to meet Dr. Alexander."

7. Performing the examination requires clear communication with the patient. You should include specific instructions about what the patient is to do next, explanations of what the radiographer is doing and reassurance that the patient is doing well. EXAMPLE: "The examination is going fine, Mrs. Davidson. We will be finished in about 3 minutes."

8. A sincere parting comment when the patient is ready to leave the department closes a very positive experience for the patient—an experience that you have successfully managed moment by moment. EXAMPLE: "Your examination is finished, Mrs. Davidson. Dr. Alexander will interpret your images and send a report to your personal physician, who I see from your chart is Dr. Mikella Jacobs. You can call Dr. Jacobs' office in a couple of days for the results. May I show you back to the dressing room? Do you know how to find the main lobby and parking area? Cara Adams at the front desk will give you a coupon for breakfast in our cafeteria. It was nice meeting you today. I hope you are feeling better soon."

The key to these interactions is that they are delivered in a sincere but timely manner. Taking too much time with one patient delivers poor service to those who are still waiting. One of your most important challenges is to deliver such value-added service in a fairly short period. Again, having total command of the technical aspects of the procedure will allow you to concentrate on patient interactions.

SERVICE ON THE TELEPHONE

Enhancing telephone interactions can play a big role in value-added service. Although most imaging departments have clerical personnel who handle many of the daily telephone calls, the radiographer is often asked to speak with inside and outside customers on the telephone. Such calls may be from patients requesting information about an examination or scheduling; physicians needing examination reports or scheduling of tests; or nursing units with questions about patient preparations, scheduling, or examinations. Each such moment of truth can reveal much about the radiographer's level of integrity, knowledge, and professionalism.

Remembering a few simple rules about using the telephone can go a long way toward improving this often-used method of communication:

1. Keep the number of rings to a minimum. If possible, answer the phone by the third ring.

2. Answer professionally. Identify the department and yourself ("Radiology. This is Troy speaking"), and add a phrase such as, "May I help you?" or "How may I help you?"

3. Enunciate carefully. Talk directly into the transmitter. Speak clearly. Do not attempt to drink, eat, or chew gum when on the telephone. Make sure your voice is pleasant and unhurried, even if you are in a hurry. Remember, you are there to assist the caller. Keep the tone of your voice alert, pleasant, and expressive. Smiling while you are speaking will automatically make your voice more pleasant. Speak more slowly than normal and with a lower voice.

4. Personalize the call. When you know the caller's name, use it. Doing so indicates a desire to assist with the request and brings the interaction to a more personal level.

5. If you have to put the caller on hold, first ask permission to do so and wait for an answer. Indicate to the caller approximately how long he or she will be waiting. When you return, thank the caller for holding. If it is necessary to put someone on hold for a long time, come back on the line about every 45 seconds to reassure the caller that the information that is needed will be available shortly.

6. Become comfortable with the telephone system quickly so that you can perform a function such as transferring a call without losing the call. If you must transfer a call, indicate the extension to which you are sending the call, and thank the caller for holding.

7. When terminating a call, thank the caller, and allow the caller to hang up first; that way you will know that the conversation has ended.

CONFLICT RESOLUTION: OPPORTUNITIES TO EXCEED PATIENT EXPECTATIONS

Leaving quality service to chance can be a serious mistake. In this age of consumer awareness and increasing competition, a mishandled patient interaction can result in the loss of patient confidence, which will reflect negatively on the department and the institution. Because of an increasingly litigious public, unprofessional interactions or mishandled complaints can increase the chances of lawsuits. Most important, exceeding patient expectations improves patient care; this is a goal to which we can all aspire. It makes radiography stimulating and satisfying for the radiographer.

Radiography is a customer-oriented business. Within this business, which is many times typified by high-stress situations and brief encounters, numerous opportunities for miscommunications and conflict exist. Other aspects of conflict are addressed in the next chapter, but the following material specifically relates to quality customer service in the radiology department. Highly successful service companies and individuals have at their disposal the **conflict resolution** tools of listening and empathizing, and they also make use of skills that build trust and develop solutions to problems. Such tools are equally useful in dealing with coworkers and physicians.

In addition, patients often have special questions for the radiographer. Being comfortable with those questions further enhances our professional standing in the eyes of the patient and increases the patient's confidence in us. Again, such interactions are not left to chance or to spur-of-the-moment answers. By anticipating questions in advance, we can have accurate, truthful, and appropriate answers ready to meet most of our patients' needs.

Most student radiographers have little or no experience in dealing with the public in the health care setting. This relationship is special and unlike any other in-service business; it provides all the more reason for thoroughly understanding basic conflict resolution early in your education program.

The first important step in conflict resolution is **effective listening** (Box 6.4). Effective listening tells others that we respect what they have to say and that we are here to help if we can. It is very important to remember that often the other person is not attacking you personally; rather, he or she is attacking a particularly unsatisfactory situation.

The second important step in conflict resolution is empathizing. **Empathy** is understanding and accepting the other person's position without necessarily agreeing or disagreeing. This can be difficult in a high-stress situation, but realizing that the person with whom you are in conflict has a right to the feelings involved is vital. Box 6.5 lists phrases that can be used when empathizing.

By empathizing with patients' feelings, you indicate a desire to respect their position and to help deal with the many emotions being expressed. Until you address the feelings, constructive problem solving cannot take place. If you diffuse the tension through listening and empathizing, then you will often find that a mutually agreeable solution is at hand.

BOX 6.4   Effective Listening Traits

Establish good eye contact with the patient (when culturally acceptable).
Face the person.
Stay physically relaxed with your arms uncrossed.
Use facial expressions to show concern.
Use vocalizations such as, "I see," and "Uh-huh."
Give your complete and undivided attention.
Avoid interrupting.

BOX 6.5   Empathetic Phrases

"I would be upset, too, if I thought ..."
"It must have been frustrating when you ..."
"I'm sorry that you are upset."
"I think I understand how you feel."
"I'm sure that was very annoying, wasn't it?"

On occasion, patients may not respond to effective listening and empathy. They may be loud and abusive or simply not interested in an agreeable solution. With such patients, you are wise to seek assistance from another radiographer, supervisor, or physician.

Listening and empathizing are also key tools to use when faced with the many questions patients may ask. As a new student radiographer, you will soon appreciate how patients feel when confronted with strange technology and uncomfortable situations. The following frequently asked patient questions and radiographer answers come from the actual experiences of student radiographers involved in patient care:

1. How much radiation am I getting?
   "With the attention radiation often gets in the media, I can understand your concern, Mr. Brown. Let me assure you that our equipment and procedures give us the information we need with a very small amount of radiation."

2. Will this hurt?
   "I can see that you are uneasy about this test, Mrs. Gonzales. There will be a little discomfort, but I will do my best to make you as comfortable as possible."

3. How much will this cost?
   "I'm sorry, but I do not know the fee for this examination. If you can wait a few moments, I will obtain the price for you, Mr. Nguyen."

4. How many pictures are you going to take?
   "I can see you are concerned about the number of images I am taking, Mrs. Makenna. It is necessary to see the area of interest from several different angles. After processing the images, I will determine if we need any additional views. We want to give you an accurate diagnosis."

5. When can I leave?
   "I'm sure that there are other things you would rather be doing, Mrs. Lightfoot. As soon as I am finished with your examination, I will see that you are released."

6. What do you see on my x-rays?
   "I'm sure that you are anxious to find out your test results, Mr. Wong. Interpreting the images is beyond my scope of practice. The radiologist will examine your images and see that your personal physician receives a copy of the results."

As you can see from these examples, a direct answer is not always possible. Many times the patient is expressing fear and anxiety; listening carefully and empathizing are excellent ways to address these feelings. Circumstances such as the concern with which a question is asked, the age of the patient, and the mental condition of the patient may certainly change how the question may be answered. No single answer will work best in every situation. Having several answers that you can use to handle different circumstances appropriately is wise.

CONCLUSION

Quality customer service is no accident. It is planned for, rehearsed, and used whenever possible. High-quality, value-added service is what the patient or customer expects, and failure to meet those expectations may send the patient elsewhere for future care. Exceeding these expectations satisfies the patient, makes your work more enjoyable, reduces stress, and benefits everyone involved. As a health care professional, you will want to deliver the best care and service possible.

QUESTIONS FOR DISCUSSION AND CRITICAL THINKING

1. Discuss experiences you have had being a patient in a hospital, clinic, or doctor's office. From your perspective as the patient, determine what interactions were positive and which were negative.

2. Based on your knowledge of your community, discuss the diversity you will likely encounter in clinical education. Decide what accommodations may be necessary to respect such diversity.

3. Visit your clinical sites' websites and view their advertising to experience how they present themselves to their patients. Evaluate how you, as a student, will need to blend with the expectations presented there.

4. Practice effective listening using the examples of empathetic statements provided.

5. Discuss the importance of properly addressing patients of various ages.

6. Discuss possible points of conflict in clinical education and how they may be managed using conflict resolution tools.

7. Reflecting on your own experiences as a patient, describe the impact of professional answers to patients' questions on their confidence in the care being provided.

8. Discuss ways in which patients define quality of care.

BIBLIOGRAPHY

Callaway W. A fresh perspective on patient care [lecture]. Springfield, IL: 2010.

Organization Dimensions. Inc: Building organizational excellence. Wheeling, IL: 1986.

Organization Dimensions. Inc: *The healthcare quality service standards system*. Wheeling, IL: 1986.

Organization Dimensions. Inc: *The quality edge*. Wheeling, IL: 1986.

Professional Research Consultants, Inc: *National consumer study*, Omaha, NE, 2017.

Salimbene S. *What language does your patient hurt in?* ed 1. St. Paul: Paradigm; 2000.

The Language of Medicine

A newcomer to the field of health care is often overwhelmed by medical terminology. As with any specialized field, the medical profession comes with a language of its own. Medical terminology is simultaneously intriguing and frustrating: the intrigue lies in the fact that you will be learning, in effect, a new language that you will use to communicate with your health care colleagues; the frustration is the same as you would experience in learning any foreign language. If you have had previous exposure to learning a second language, then medical terminology may come easily to you. If not, this learning experience will be an exciting new endeavor, although it may be somewhat confusing because of the unfamiliar combinations of word parts used to form the medical vocabulary.

Everyone working in health care should know relevant medical terminology. Each medical specialty, including radiologic technology, has its unique terms. Both general and specific terminologies are covered in this chapter, but exploring the entire collection of terms that you will need to learn is not possible. Early exposure to this nomenclature, however, will greatly aid in your understanding of the language you will soon hear. As with any foreign language, the best method for first learning the material is memorization.

As you study the words and combining forms in this chapter, keep in mind that most of them are of Latin or Greek origin. To those who have spoken English since childhood, the relationship between these words and the concepts they represent may seem questionable. A student who is interested in an in-depth study of medical terminology can refer to any reputable medical dictionary or terminology textbook (print or electronic) for further information about the words presented in this chapter.

WORD PARTS

The following section introduces the word parts that are used to make new words; these parts include **prefixes**, **roots**, and **suffixes**. They are presented in alphabetical order in each category (Box 7.1).

BOX 7.1   Word Parts

Prefixes

ab-	away from
a-, an-	without
ante-	front
anti-	against
bi-	two
co-	together
contra-	against
decub-	side
dors-	back
dys-	difficult
ect-	outside
en-	in
endo-	within
epi-	upon
ex-	out
hemi-	half
hydro-	water
hyper-	above or greater
hypo-	below or lesser
infero-	below
megal-	large
pan-	all
peri-	around
poly-	many
post-	back, after
pre-	before
pseudo-	false
retro-	backward
scler-	hard
sub-	below
super-	above
trans-	across
tri-	three
vent-	front

Roots

angio	vessel
arth	joint
cardi	heart
cephal	brain
cerebro	head
cerv	neck
chiro	hand
enter	intestine
gastr	stomach
hem	blood
hepat	liver
hyster	uterus
leuk	white
lith	stone

Suffixes

-algia	pain
-centesis	puncture
-dia	through
-ectomy	excision
-emia	blood
-ectasis	expansion
-genic	origin
-iasis	condition
-itis	inflammation
-megaly	enlargement
-myel	spinal cord
-oid	like
-oma	tumor
-osis	condition
-pathy	disease
-plasty	surgical correction
-pulm	lung
-pyel	pelvis (renal)
-rhaphy	suture
-scopy	inspection
-tomy	incision

MEDICAL ABBREVIATIONS

Abbreviations are as much a part of medical communication as words. The following list contains the most common abbreviations that you may encounter during examination requisitions, on surgery schedules, and in patients' charts or electronic medical record (EMR):

AIDS	acquired immunodeficiency syndrome
ARC	AIDS-related complex
ASAP	as soon as possible
ASHD	arteriosclerotic heart disease
BE	barium enema
BID	twice daily
BP	blood pressure
BUN	blood urea nitrogen
Bx	biopsy
c̄	with
CA	cancer

CAD	coronary artery disease		LBP	low back pain
CBC	complete blood count		LMP	last menstrual period
cc	cubic centimeter		LLQ	left lower quadrant (of the abdomen)
CCU	coronary care unit		LUP	left upper quadrant (of the abdomen)
CE, CEU	continuing education, continuing education unit		mets	metastases
			MI	myocardial infarction (heart attack)
CHF	congestive heart failure		mm	millimeter
cm	centimeter		MRI; MR	magnetic resonance imaging
CNS	central nervous system		MRSA	methicillin-resistant *Staphylococcus aureus*
C/O	complains of		MVA	motor vehicle accident
COPD	chronic obstructive pulmonary disease		NG	nasogastric
CPR	cardiopulmonary resuscitation		NICU	neonatal intensive care unit
CS	central supply		noc	night
C-section	cesarean section		npo	nothing by mouth
CSF	cerebrospinal fluid		OB	obstetrics
CT	computed tomography		OP	outpatient
CVA	cerebrovascular accident (stroke)		OR	operating room
CXR	chest x-ray		OTC	over the counter
DNR	do not resuscitate order, no code		PACU	postanesthesia care unit
DOA	dead on arrival		PE	physical examination
DOB	date of birth		peds	pediatrics
DX	diagnosis		PID	pelvic inflammatory disease
ECG; EKG	electrocardiogram		p/o	postoperative
EEG	electroencephalogram		post-OP	after surgery
EMG	electromyogram		pre-OP	before surgery
EMR	electronic medical record		prn	as needed
ENT	ear, nose, and throat		PT	physical therapy; prothrombin time
ER; ED	emergency room; emergency department		pt	patient
FB	foreign body		PTSD	post-traumatic stress disorder
FUO	fever of undetermined origin		QID	four times daily
Fx	fracture		R/O	rule out
GI	gastrointestinal		req	requisition
GSW	gunshot wound		RLQ	right lower quadrant (of the abdomen)
HH	hiatal hernia		ROM	range of motion
HHS	United States Department of Health and Human Services		RUQ	right upper quadrant (of the abdomen)
			Rx	treatment or prescription
HIPAA	Health Insurance Portability and Accountability Act of 1996		s̄	without
			SIDS	sudden infant death syndrome
HIV	human immunodeficiency virus		SOB	short of breath
H/O	history of		S/P	status post (after)
Hx	history		STAT	immediately
IBD	inflammatory bowel disease		STD	sexually transmitted disease
IBS	inflammatory bowel syndrome		Sx	symptoms
ICCU	intensive coronary care unit		TB	tuberculosis
ICU	intensive care unit		TIA	transient ischemic attack
IM	intramuscular		TID	three times daily
I/O	intake and output		TKO	to keep open (refers to IV line)
IV	intravenous		TPN	total parenteral nutrition (IV feeding)
IVP, IVU	intravenous pyelogram, intravenous urogram		TPR	temperature, pulse, and respiration
			Tx	treatment
KUB	kidneys, ureters, and bladder		UA	urinalysis
lat	lateral		UGI	upper gastrointestinal series

URI	upper respiratory infection
UTI	urinary tract infection
VD	venereal disease
VSS	vital signs stable
y/o	years old

TITLES AND ORGANIZATIONS

You will be seeing and hearing the abbreviations for various titles and the names of organizations in the literature you read and in use throughout the hospital. The following list contains many that you will encounter:

ACERT	Association of Collegiate Educators in Radiologic Technology
ACR	American College of Radiology
AEIRS	Association of Educators in Imaging and Radiologic Sciences
AHA	American Hospital Association
AHRA	The Association for Medical Imaging Management
AMA	American Medical Association
ANA	American Nurses Association
ARDMS	American Registry of Diagnostic Medical Sonographers
ARRT	American Registry of Radiologic Technologists
ASRT	American Society of Radiologic Technologists
CDC	Centers for Disease Control and Prevention
CNA	certified nursing assistant
EAP	employee assistance program
EMT	emergency medical technician
HMO	health maintenance organization
ISRRT	International Society of Radiographers and Radiologic Technologists
JRCERT	Joint Review Committee on Education in Radiologic Technology
LPN	licensed practical nurse
MD	medical doctor; physician
MT	medical technologist
NCRP	National Council on Radiation Protection and Measurements
NIH	National Institutes of Health
NMTCB	Nuclear Medicine Technology Certification Board
OSHA	Occupational Safety and Health Administration
PA	physician assistant
PPO	preferred provider organization
RDMS	Registered Diagnostic Medical Sonographer
RN	registered nurse
RPH	registered pharmacist
RPT	registered physical therapist

RRA	registered radiologist assistant
RRT	registered respiratory therapist
RSNA	Radiological Society of North America
RT(BD)	Registered Technologist in Bone Densitometry
RT(BS)	Registered Technologist in Breast Sonography
RT(CI)	Registered Technologist in Cardiac Interventional Radiography
RT(CT)	Registered Technologist in Computed Tomography
RT(M)	Registered Technologist in Mammography
RT(MR)	Registered Technologist in Magnetic Resonance Imaging
RT(N)	Registered Technologist in Nuclear Medicine
RT(R)	Registered Technologist in Radiography
RT(S)	Registered Technologist in Sonography
RT(T)	Registered Technologist in Radiation Therapy
RT(VI)	Registered Technologist in Vascular Interventional Radiography
RT(VS)	Registered Technologist in Vascular Sonography
SDMS	Society of Diagnostic Medical Sonographers
SI	international system of units
SMRI	Society of Magnetic Resonance Imaging
SNM	Society of Nuclear Medicine
TJC	The Joint Commission
WHO	World Health Organization

RADIOGRAPHIC NOMENCLATURE

Terms relating to your chosen specialty are of paramount importance if you are to function comfortably in the clinical setting. The following list contains the most common terms that you will need to know:

ADC (analog-to-digital converter)   converts image information into numerical data

AEC automatic exposure control (ionization chamber located between the patient and the image receptor)

algorithm mathematical formula used by the computer to construct the radiographic image

anode positive electrode in the x-ray tube

APR; APT anatomically programmed radiography; anatomically programmed technique; exposure technique is set by the radiographer by choosing the proper anatomic part and projection on the control panel

artifact an unwanted marking on a radiographic image

automatic collimation also known as positive beam limitation (PBL); the ability of the radiographic equipment to collimate automatically the x-ray beam to the same size as the image receptor resting in the Bucky tray

bit binary digit either 1 or 0; the computer's unit of information

bit depth the number of shades of gray available within a pixel

blur effect of motion on the radiographic image

brightness, image brightness the amount of light coming from the monitor on which the radiographic image is displayed

Bucky short for Potter-Bucky diaphragm; a moving grid used to remove scatter radiation from the remnant beam, which can cause fog on the image receptor

cassette container used for holding the imaging plate in computed radiography (CR)

cathode negative electrode in the x-ray tube

collimator box-like structure attached to the x-ray tube containing lead shutters that limit the x-ray beam to a specific area of the body

contrast media solutions or gasses introduced into the body to increase the scale of contrast, making more detail visible; negative contrast medium is air; positive contrast media are barium and iodine

computed radiography (CR) digital radiographic imaging using a cassette containing an imaging plate

contrast the visible difference between two selected areas of brightness in the radiographic image; contrast allows detail to be visible

contrast resolution the smallest change in signal that can be detected by the image receptor

DAP dose area product, a measure of the total radiation exposure to the patient, extrapolated from the dose in the air just above the patient

DICOM (digital imaging and communications in medicine) a standard protocol used for blending a picture archiving and communications system and various imaging modalities

direct radiography (DR) uses fixed detectors that directly communicate with a computer

distortion misrepresentation of the size or shape of the object as recorded in the radiographic image

dynamic range the ability of an image receptor to capture the x-ray photons leaving the patient

exposure indicator describes the status of the exposure and diagnostic value of the digital image

fluoroscopy "live action" imaging when the x-ray beam is on, creating images of the body as it functions and displaying those images on a monitor

focal spot (focal track) area of the anode in the x-ray tube from which x-rays emanate

grid device that is placed between the patient and the image receptor that absorbs scatter radiation exiting the body

HIS hospital information system

HL7 health level seven, an international standard for communicating medical information

histogram graphic display of the distribution of pixel values in a digital image

image receptor (IR) any device or medium that captures the remnant beam

imaging plate (IP) plate that is coated with photostimulable phosphors that absorb the photon energies exiting the patient; located inside a computed radiography (CR) cassette

kVp peak kilovoltage that is applied to the x-ray tube, which determines the wavelength of the x-ray beam and its ability to penetrate the body, impacting the overall contrast of the radiographic image

lead aprons coverings worn by radiographers who are in a radiographic or fluoroscopic room with the x-ray beam turned on; also required to be worn for radiation protection when performing portable radiography; the lead absorbs most of the scatter radiation that strikes the apron

mAs (milliampere-seconds) the product of milliamperage and time; mA is the current that is passed through the x-ray tube, whose energy is then converted to x-rays when it strikes the anode; it determines the number of x-rays produced and, consequently, the overall exposure striking the image receptor; radiation exposure to the patient is directly proportional to the mAs used

matrix digital image that is made up of rows and columns of data

mobile radiography, portable radiography imaging patients in locations other than an x-ray room, such as the patient's room or operating room (see surgical radiography); because of presence of scatter radiation, the radiographer is required to wear a dosimeter and lead apron

OID (object-to-image receptor distance) distance from the part being examined to the image receptor

PACS picture archiving and communications system

pixel picture element; the smallest component of a matrix

postprocessing digital manipulation of a radiographic image after its acquisition by the computer

PSP (photostimulable phosphor) coating on the imaging plate of a computed radiography cassette

radiographic image x-ray image as viewed on a monitor after acquisition

radiographic position specific position of the body or body part in relation to the table or image receptor

radiographic projection path the x-ray beam takes as it passes through the body; described as if the body is in the anatomical position

radiographic view term used to explain how the image receptor sees the body image; the opposite of the radiographic projection

remnant beam (exit radiation) x-ray beam that exits the patient; is made up of image-forming rays and scatter radiation

RIS radiology information system

scatter radiation x-rays emanating from the patient in divergent paths rather than straight to the image receptor; the source of the radiographer's occupational dose, requiring the wearing of a lead apron and dosimeter for fluoroscopy and mobile radiography

spatial resolution the sharpness of the structural edges in the radiographic image; the smallest detail that can be detected

SID (source-to-image receptor distance) distance from the source of radiation (x-ray tube anode) to the image receptor

SOD (source-to-object distance) distance from the source of radiation (x-ray tube anode) to the part being examined

surgical radiography radiographic procedures performed by the radiographer in the operating room, usually using a C-arm (portable fluoroscope)

time, distance, shielding the three cardinal principles of radiation protection; least amount of time exposed, greatest distance from the source of radiation, use of lead or other barriers to shield

voxel volume element; section of tissue represented by a pixel

window level midpoint of densities in a digital image; used to adjust digital image brightness

window width adjusts contrast of the digital image

workstation (radiologist or radiographer) location of the monitor on which radiographic images are displayed

x-ray a form of electromagnetic radiation at wavelengths that can penetrate matter

INAPPROPRIATE OR UNACCEPTABLE ABBREVIATIONS

Only standardized abbreviations may be used in health care settings. This chapter, along with a comprehensive course in medical terminology, serves as a guide to the acceptable abbreviations used. The Joint Commission (TJC) maintains an official list of abbreviations and symbols, along with acronyms, that may *not* be used in health care communication. Be certain to visit the website at http://www.jointcommission.org/patientsafety/donotuselist for the most current listing and be very familiar with its content.

CONCLUSION

Many other terms relating to radiography will be presented in appropriate classes during the course of your education. This listing is by no means complete, but it will give you a good start as you begin your studies. To assist with your comprehension of this material, complete the exercises at the end of this chapter.

QUESTIONS FOR DISCUSSION AND CRITICAL THINKING

1. Discuss the importance of learning the language of medicine.
2. Explain the advantages of all medical personnel speaking the same professional language.
3. Some terminology is unique to radiology. Discuss why it is important to master these terms before entering the clinical setting.

BIBLIOGRAPHY

Bushong S. *Radiologic science for technologists.* ed 11. St. Louis: Elsevier; 2017.

American Registry of Radiologic Technologists, Available at http://www.arrt.org.

Callaway W. *Mosby's comprehensive review of radiography.* ed 7. St. Louis: Elsevier; 2017.

Fauber T. *Radiographic imaging & exposure.* ed 5. St. Louis: Elsevier; 2017.

Johnston J, Fauber T. *Essentials of radiographic physics and imaging.* ed 2. St. Louis: Elsevier; 2016.

Long B, Rollins J, Smith B. *Merrill's atlas of radiographic positioning and procedures.* ed 14. St. Louis: Elsevier; 2019.

8

The Technology of Medical Imaging

OBJECTIVES

On completion of this chapter, you should be able to:

- Describe the x-ray tube and name its two main components.
- Explain the basic process of x-ray production.
- Discuss the use of direct digital radiography.
- Explain the role of mAs and kVp in image production.
- Describe the image characteristics of image brightness, contrast, spatial resolution, and distortion.
- Describe the function of the fluoroscope.
- Explain the advantage to using computed tomography.
- Explain how an image is made in nuclear medicine.
- Describe the use of portable radiographic and fluoroscopic units.
- Discuss how an image is formed in sonography.
- List the two types of information obtained by using magnetic resonance imaging.
- Explain the primary use of positron emission computed tomography.
- Discuss the technologist's role in image production and evaluation.
- Explain the use of the picture archiving and communication system in radiographic imaging.

CHAPTER OUTLINE

X-Ray Tube
Radiographic Imaging
Factors Affecting the Image
  Subject Density and Thickness
  X-Ray Exposure Factors
Characteristics of the Radiographic Image
  Image Brightness
  Image Contrast
  Spatial Resolution
  Distortion

Other Imaging Technology
  Fluoroscopy
  Computed Tomography
  Magnetic Resonance Imaging
  Nuclear Medicine
  Positron Emission Tomography
  Portable Radiography and Fluoroscopy
  Diagnostic Medical Sonography
  Picture Archiving and Communication System
Conclusion

KEY TERMS

anode
cathode
collimator
computed tomography (CT)
contrast media
density
detail
diagnostic medical sonography
digital communications in medicine (DICOM)
direct digital radiography

distortion
elongation
fluoroscopy
fog
foreshortening
grids
hospital information system (HIS)
image brightness
image contrast
image intensifier
image receptor (IR)

kilovoltage (kVp)
magnetic resonance imaging (MRI)
magnification
milliampere-seconds (mAs)
nuclear medicine
object-to-image receptor distance (OID)
picture archiving and communication system (PACS)
portable radiography and fluoroscopy

Accurately imaging the human body is the goal of medical radiography. In-depth knowledge of the equipment is essential for making proper exposures and acquiring diagnostic images. Such studies are covered in detail in equipment and imaging courses. This chapter summarizes the types of equipment used in imaging to help you understand what you will be seeing early in your educational program.

After a physician has determined the need for radiographic studies and orders an examination, the radiographer is responsible for obtaining the best possible diagnostic images. The technologist evaluates the orders from the physician and greets the patient in the imaging department. Establishing a cordial relationship with the patient helps the radiographer obtain the needed diagnostic examination. Patient interaction is discussed at length in Chapter 6.

The anatomic part to be radiographed will be positioned and evaluated to determine the thickness of the part and the overall tissue **density**. Then, when the image is acquired, it must be examined for diagnostic quality (Figure 8.1, *A, B, C*). Basic x-ray equipment and image characteristics are discussed in the following sections.

X-RAY TUBE

X-rays are not stored, nor do they come from radioactive materials. The radiographer creates an x-ray beam for each exposure using technical factors manipulated on the x-ray control panel. X-rays are produced by a series of energy conversions. The primary items needed for the production of x-rays are (1) a source of electrons, (2) a means to accelerate the electrons, and (3) a way to bring the electrons to a sudden stop. All of this takes place in the x-ray tube.

The **x-ray tube** is an evacuated glass bulb with positive (anode) and negative (cathode) electrodes (Figure 8.2). The **cathode** is a filament that gives off electrons when heated (i.e., the source of electrons). As several thousand volts of electricity are applied across the tube, these electrons are driven across a short distance at a very high speed (i.e., the means to accelerate the electrons) and strike the anode with high kinetic energy (i.e., the way to bring the electrons to a sudden stop). The **anode** is the electrode the electrons strike. It is a metal disc made of a high atomic number metal. Because energy can be neither created nor destroyed, an energy conversion takes place; this energy conversion is the result of the sudden deceleration of the electrons at the anode. Heat is the primary by-product (>99%) of this energy conversion. However, x-rays are also produced (<1%), and they emanate from the anode in all directions, travelling at the speed of light, which is 186,000 miles per second. The x-rays exit the tube housing through a device consisting of open lead shutters called a **collimator**. The collimator permits the radiographer to determine the size of the exposure field on the patient.

RADIOGRAPHIC IMAGING

Substantial increases in the speed of computer microprocessors, combined with relatively inexpensive memory and large storage capability, account for the complete use of digital medical imaging.

Digital imaging equipment enhances images of the body. The primary advantages of digital equipment include speed of image acquisition and the ability to postprocess images in a variety of ways to provide multiple characteristics of the anatomy. Characteristics of the image can be altered any time after the completion of the study without re-exposing the patient. The images are stored in memory and can be transferred to multiple locations on a network or sent via e-mail.

Direct digital radiography (DR), as it is called, uses an imaging plate (IP) that remains in place inside the x-ray table or wall unit. The IP is also known as the **image receptor (IR)**. The DR image appears on the monitor almost immediately after exposure. A separate moveable DR plate is used for portable radiography.

Storing images for future review and comparison is a significant advantage to DR. The images can be stored on servers and retrieved for review at a later date.

Given a wide range in exposure latitude, retakes can be greatly reduced because the image can be altered without further exposure to the patient. A word of caution is required here. Being able to manipulate the image is a mixed blessing. Some radiographers may be careless with the exposure factors and overexpose, giving the patient more radiation than is necessary, knowing the image can be adjusted. Dr. Terri Fauber has conducted extensive research on radiation exposure and digital imaging. She reminds radiographers that "overexposing patients is an objectionable practice" (Fauber, 2009). Digital imaging will tolerate a range of error in exposure technique, but proper technical factors are critical in protecting the patient from

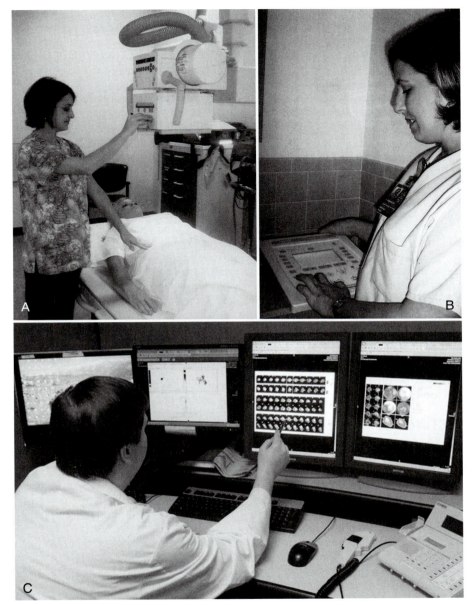

Fig. 8.1 A, Positioning of the patient is critical. The anatomy of interest must be imaged for diagnostic interpretation. **B,** Exposure factors that affect the diagnostic quality of images are selected at the control panel. **C,** Radiographic image is interpreted. (*Part A,* Courtesy of Amy Justice Hill, University of Mississippi Medical Center. *Part B,* Courtesy of technologist Tamara Rodriguez, University of Mississippi Medical Center. *Part C,* Courtesy of Colin Wentworth and Methodist University Hospital; Joseph Martin, photographer.)

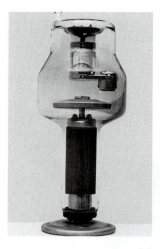

Fig. 8.2 A typical x-ray tube shows cathode *(top)* and anode *(bottom)* within the glass envelope.

unwanted or unnecessary radiation. All radiographers must keep the exposure to the patient as low as reasonably achievable (ALARA).[a]

This chapter discusses several factors that affect the production of a radiographic image. For every concept briefly discussed in this text, a substantial amount of theory and practical application will be presented in the classroom and in your clinical experience.

FACTORS AFFECTING THE IMAGE

Subject Density and Thickness

The density of tissues is primarily a matter of the atomic number of the elements making up the tissues. Bone, which is made up of calcium (atomic number 20), phosphorus (atomic number 15), and other elements, has an average atomic number of approximately 14. However, soft tissue, which is mostly water, has an average atomic number of 7.5. The atomic number does not tell the whole story because the average atomic number of air and soft issues is about the same. Yet because air is a gas, it obeys the law of gases

and fills a container; thus, air molecules are not as tightly packed as water molecules. Another example is ice, which is frozen water with the same atomic number as water; however, it is approximately 9% less dense than water because of the molecular arrangement.

The human body consists of six radiographic densities. The following list is in order of the least dense to the most dense:

1. Air or gas, which is present in such areas as the lungs, stomach, and intestines
2. Fat, which surrounds abdominal organs and the abdominal wall, as well as being a factor when radiographing obese patients
3. Water, present in all cells and accumulating in severe sprains
4. Muscle, which contains large amounts of water and has approximately the same density as the heart and blood vessels
5. Bone, which is denser than other tissues, except when affected by osteoporosis
6. Tooth enamel, the densest tissue in the body

Metal is a non-naturally occurring density, which is encountered in radiography in several ways:

1. Foreign bodies such as bullets, swallowed articles, or items inserted into the body
2. Prostheses such as metallic nails, screws, and pins used to align fractured bones as well as artificial hips, knees, and other anatomy
3. Contrast media such as barium, which is a metallic salt, and iodine. Although it is a non-metal, iodine shares some properties with metals
4. Cardiac pacemakers and the associated wires
5. Jewelry, piercings, and so on

Furthermore, other non-naturally occurring densities encountered in radiography may be dental prostheses, implants, and supporting plates.

Each density presents a difference in the degree of absorption of radiation. Gas is less dense than fat and thus absorbs less radiation than fat, muscle, or bone. Figure 8.3 illustrates various radiographic appearances.

The thickness of the part to be examined also influences the absorption of radiation. With all other factors remaining the same, the thicker the part, the greater the radiation absorption. This is particularly important when radiographing injuries that cause swelling, such as severe sprains, as well as the rapidly growing issue of obesity in the population.

The age of the patient, the patient's lifestyle, and the patient's state of health each play a part in the texture, structure, and condition of the tissue. A disease may be demonstrated as a more or less dense area as compared with the adjacent healthy tissue.

---

[a]In another type of digital imaging known as computed radiography (CR), x-rays exit the patient and strike a cassette containing an imaging plate. The IP is coated with a substance known as a *photostimulable phosphor*. This phosphor becomes excited as a result of the deposit of x-ray energy, and it remains so until the cassette is placed in a reader. When inside the reader, the IP is scanned with a laser beam, releasing the x-ray energy that is then converted to a visible image by the computer. The resulting image is viewed on a monitor. Although currently used in a number of clinical settings, CR is rapidly being replaced by DR.

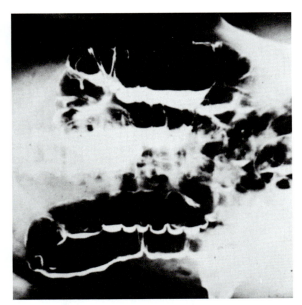

Fig. 8.3 Radiographic image shows the radiographic densities of gas (or air), fat, muscle, and bone. The fifth density, the metallic contrast medium barium, is shown in this air-barium, double-contrast colon study. Note: The heavy barium gravitates to the lower level; the lightweight air rises to the top.

X-Ray Exposure Factors

With the typical x-ray machine, the primary controls to be adjusted are **milliampere-seconds (mAs)** and **kilovoltage (kVp)**. mAs determines, the current, or flow of electrons, for a certain length of time, normally thousandths of a second. kVp, or kilovolts-peak, determines the "force" behind the flow of electrons and is the factor that determines the penetrating ability of the radiation It affects the energy of the radiation that will go deep into the tissues and through the patient to strike the image receptor. Radiation produced at low-voltage settings is weak in energy and may be stopped or absorbed in the first few centimeters of tissue.

With these three factors in mind—amperage, time, and voltage—you can learn to adjust them for the desired results. In most cases, you will use anatomically programmed radiography (APR) to set the technique based on the part being radiographed. However, it is very important to still be able to set or vary radiographic exposure manually for variations in anatomy, pathology, or trauma.

Milliampere-Seconds

The x-ray exposure rate is directly proportional to milliamperage because milliamperage determines the amount of x-rays produced per unit of time. With all factors remaining the same, the greater the mAs, the greater the

amount of radiation produced. If the mAs is halved, the amount of x-rays is reduced by half. Thus the amount of remnant radiation striking the image receptor is directly proportional to the mAs.

Kilovoltage

Kilovoltage has an effect on imaging because it determines the wavelength of the x-rays produced and thus the beam's penetrating power; the greater the penetrating ability of the x-rays, the greater the amount of remnant radiation reaching the image receptor. As discussed earlier, the higher the kilovoltage, the greater the energy of the radiation; consequently, more x-rays traverse the patient and strike the receptor. Kilovoltage, combined with the atomic number of the anatomical parts, controls the differential absorption of the x-ray beam in the body. This results in contrast on the image, which allows detail to be visible.

Distance

Distance as discussed here relates to the distance from the radiation source (x-ray tube) to the image receptor. X-rays emerge from the tube, diverge, and proceed in straight paths. Because of the divergence, they cover an increasingly large area as they travel farther away from the tube. The radiation emitted from the tube remains the same; however, because a larger area is covered as the distance increases, the amount of radiation per square inch is reduced.

The decrease in the amount of radiation at a greater distance is solely a geometric factor relating to the divergent x-ray beam (Figure 8.4). The absorption of x-rays by intervening air is insignificant and can be totally disregarded.

CHARACTERISTICS OF THE RADIOGRAPHIC IMAGE

Image Brightness

The **image brightness,** or the brightness of the radiographic image, is the amount of light emission from the computer monitor. Areas of greater brightness correspond to less dense areas of the body, and areas of lesser brightness demonstrate denser regions of anatomy. This is determined by the intensity of radiation striking the image receptor, called receptor exposure. The quality of the image is determined by the appropriate receptor exposure, controlled by kVp and mAs.

Image Contrast

Image contrast may be defined as the visible difference between two areas of brightness in the displayed image. Brightness and contrast are discussed as if they are separate properties, but the definition of contrast reminds us they

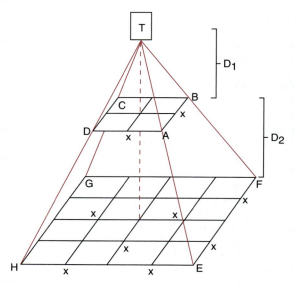

Fig. 8.4 Divergent rays increase the area covered. The diagram shows the lower surface area four times the size of the upper surface area because it is twice the distance from the x-ray source.

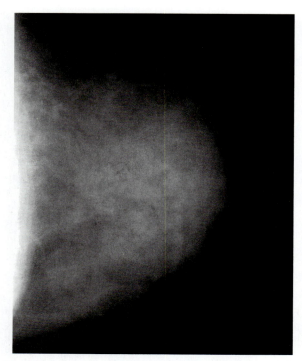

Fig. 8.5 Breast tissue has little subject contrast because of the small variations in the atomic number of the structures.

combine to create an image. From the standpoint of exposure, contrast is controlled by kVp because of its control of the differential absorption of the x-ray beam by the body. **Subject contrast**, that is, the patient's anatomy, also plays a major role in determining the overall contrast on the image (Figure 8.5). Software may be used postexposure to alter the overall scale of contrast in the image.

In imaging, one can also speak of contrast resolution, which is the smallest change in signal detected by the image receptor.

Furthermore, **contrast media** affect contrast because they have different radiation-absorbing properties. For example, barium and iodine, which have high atomic numbers, absorb relatively more radiation than the adjacent tissues and thus increase contrast. Air, which is less dense than tissue and absorbs less radiation than adjacent tissues, also improves contrast, proving again that the absorption differences of structures and materials greatly affect contrast.

Fog

Fog from any source, though primarily scatter radiation emanating from the patient, increases the overall darkness of the radiographic image. The density produced by fog does not add to the diagnostic quality of the image; rather, it detracts from the quality because the overall grayness obliterates small structures that are beneficial to its

diagnostic quality. Fog increases as the volume of tissue increases. In the case of a skull radiograph (Figure 8.6, *A*), the image is so overcast with fog that its diagnostic quality is unacceptable.

When the field size is reduced to a small volume of tissue (Figure 8.6, *B*), fog reduces dramatically. Collimators are beam-limiting devices attached to the x-ray tube to reduce exposure field size. They decrease the amount of radiation striking the patient because they reduce the overall area of the x-ray beam. Thus, there is a decrease in the amount of scatter radiation produced. Scatter radiation decreases as the volume of irradiated tissue decreases.

Grids are used to absorb scatter radiation before it reaches the image receptor (Figure 8.7). By preventing scatter radiation from striking the image receptor, the overall contrast of the image is improved. Since scatter and some of the image forming rays are absorbed by grids, receptor exposure is decreased.

Spatial Resolution

The ability to see **detail** in an image is often called visibility of detail. It is controlled by the contrast present in the image. The interaction between the x-ray beam (kVp)

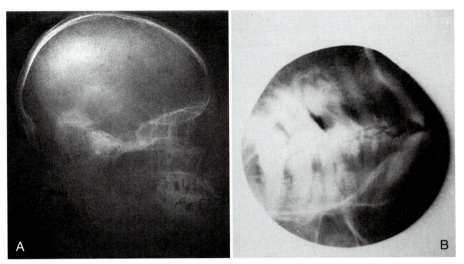

Fig. 8.6 A, Radiograph made without the use of a beam-limiting device. **B,** Radiograph made with a beam-limiting device. Note: Scatter radiation is reduced with a decrease of tissue volume.

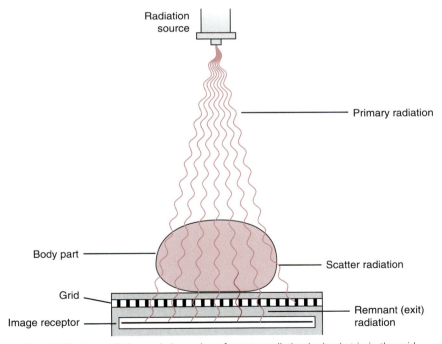

Fig. 8.7 Scatter radiation and absorption of scatter radiation by lead strip in the grid.

and the patient's tissues determines contrast. Without contrast, detail cannot be seen.

Spatial resolution may be thought of as the sharpness of the structures in the radiographic image. From the viewpoint of the radiologist who is interpreting the image, detail is the crux of image quality and thus is first in importance. The size and spacing of pixels in the image receptor play a role in optimal spatial resolution. These are not, however, controlled by the radiographer and are instead characteristic of the brand of image receptor being used. Likewise, the focal spot size in the x-ray tube also impacts resolution but is generally not controlled by the radiographer in modern x-ray equipment.

However, the radiographer does control other factors controlling resolution. These are **source-to-image receptor distance (SID)**, **object-to-image receptor distance (OID)**, and motion. Higher resolution occurs when using the longest practical SID and the lowest practical OID.

X-radiation can be compared to visible light in that x-rays follow many of the rules that govern the formation of shadows by light. A familiar observation is the shadow cast in the surface of a plane at some distance from a light source; the nearer a hand is to the plane's surface, the sharper the edges of the silhouette. As the hand moves farther away from the plane's surface, the more indistinct the edges of the shadow become. To improve the sharpness of the image (and thereby enhance detail), the anatomic part of interest should be placed as near to the receptor as possible (Figure 8.8). The same geometry applies to SID. These situations can be easily demonstrated using a flashlight, a hand, and a blank wall and varying the distance between the flashlight, the hand, and the wall.

In most cases, these distances are standardized for nearly all examinations. However, mobile radiography can present a challenge. The radiographer must keep in

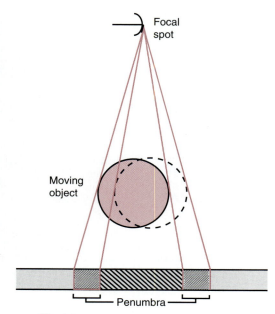

Fig. 8.9 Effects of motion on unsharpness.

mind the impact of SID and OID on image resolution in those cases.

Motion, either patient or equipment, can destroy spatial resolution very easily. Patient motion is perhaps the greatest factor encountered that affects detail in medical imaging. Breathing or otherwise moving during the exposure causes blurring of the image; consequently, detail is greatly impaired (Figure 8.9). Although not as common, vibration of the x-ray tube at the moment of exposure also affects detail. This could result from excessive pressing of the positioning light button on an x-ray tube or instability of the locks on a portable x-ray machine.

Distortion

Image **distortion** is a false representation of the object being radiographed. Factors that may contribute to distortion are SID, OID, and beam alignment.

The two types of image distortion are size and shape. Size distortion is **magnification**, making the part appear larger than it really is. Size distortion occurs from using too short of an SID or too long of an OID. Optimal SID should always be used. Shortest OID, by placing the part as close to the image receptor as possible, should be used.

Shape distortion can take two forms, **foreshortening** and **elongation**. Whereas foreshortening makes the object appear shorter than it is, elongation makes the object appear longer than it is. Shape distortion is caused by inappropriate angling of the x-ray tube or part being

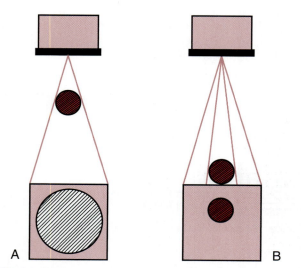

Fig. 8.8 A, The object being radiographed is magnified in the image because of its distance from the image receptor. **B,** The object is near the image receptor, and little magnification is present.

radiographed. Angling the tube against the long-axis of the part results in the anatomy appearing shorter than it is by superimposing part of the anatomy upon itself. Angling the tube along the long-axis of the part will cause it to appear longer than is actually is. Similarly, rotating or angling the part results in shape distortion as well.

For proper visual representation of anatomy in a radiographic image, the x-ray tube, part, and image receptor must be in parallel planes. Although this is not usually a problem in "routine" examinations, it can become an issue when performing mobile radiography or radiographing patients remaining on a cart. The radiographer must use special care and take extra precautions so as to not introduce distortion into a radiographic image (Figure 8.10). As you will learn in later coursework, some radiographic projections purposely use distortion to better visualize certain body parts.

Beam alignment relates to the alignment of the object in relation to the x-ray tube and image receptor, which in turn determines the shape as seen in the radiographic image. For example, an oval object will be imaged as a circle (Figure 8.11, A), and a rectangular object will be imaged as a square (Figure 8.11, B). The oil in water that has risen to the top with the x-ray beam directed downward is not discernible. Only when the tube is directed to be horizontal to the object can the difference in densities be seen (Figure 8.12).

If the long axes of these objects are placed at right angles to the direction of the beam and parallel to the image receptor, the images will be shown in another perspective. They can then be identified by their actual geometric shape.

OTHER IMAGING TECHNOLOGY

Fluoroscopy

Certain examinations in radiology make use of **fluoroscopy**, which provides a *live-action* view of the interior of the body. In fluoroscopy, the x-ray tube in most installations is located inside the x-ray table. The radiation passes through the tabletop and the patient, and it strikes the **image intensifier** tube or flat panel detector, which electronically brightens and enhances the image and transmits it to the monitor. Usually the radiologist operates the fluoroscopy unit while the radiographer assists with the patient and the procedure. If the radiologist wants to make a permanent record of the image, digital fluoroscopy allows an image to be captured, saved in a computer, and postprocessed in a variety of ways.

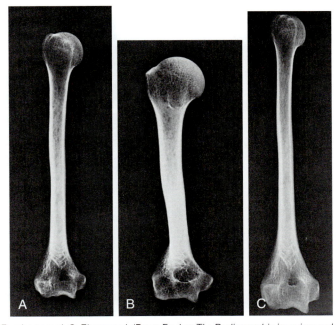

Fig. 8.10 A, No distortion. **B,** Forshortened. **C,** Elongated. (From Fauber TL: *Radiographic imaging and exposure*, ed 5, St. Louis, 2017, Elsevier.)

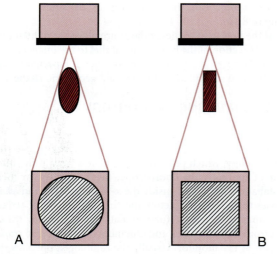

Fig. 8.11 A, Radiograph of an oval object may appear as a circle. **B,** Radiograph of a rectangular object may appear as a square.

Computed Tomography

Computed tomography (CT) units provide cross-sectional views of the body. This imaging equipment greatly improves the accuracy of diagnoses and greatly reduces the need for exploratory surgery. With the patient lying on a movable couch, an x-ray tube and a radiation detector rotate around the table; this rotation provides the computer with a *slab* of information about the patient's body. The computer reconstructs the information into an image that is viewed on a monitor and stored for later retrieval and interpretation. CT scanners are able to obtain several dozen *slices* of information with one exposure. CT is a routine imaging device used extensively in radiography.

Magnetic Resonance Imaging

Magnetic resonance imaging (MRI) units allow cross-sectional views of the body to be made without the use of ionizing radiation. With the patient lying on the couch in the cylindrical imager, the body part in question is exposed to a magnetic field and radio wave transmission. The images are produced in the computer by reconstructing the information that was received from the interaction of

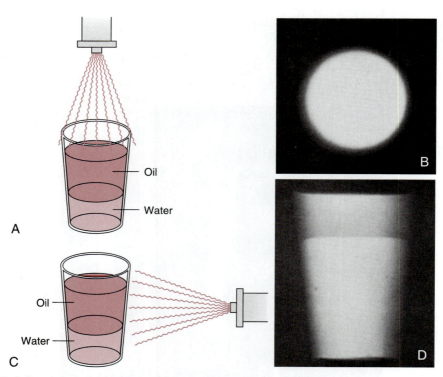

Fig. 8.12 A, Drawing of oil on water with the x-ray beam directed vertically. **B,** Radiograph of oil on water with the x-ray beam directed vertically. **C,** Drawing of oil on water with the x-ray beam directed horizontally. **D,** Radiograph of oil on water with the x-ray beam directed horizontally.

radio waves and magnetism with the body part. The information and images provide the physician with data about both the anatomy and the physiologic characteristics of the body part being examined.

Nuclear Medicine

In **nuclear medicine**, radiopharmaceuticals introduced into the body are used to produce images of major organs. The radioactive material concentrates in the area of interest and emits radiation; this radiation is then detected by a sensing device and is computed into an image.

Positron Emission Tomography

Positron emission tomography (PET) is similar to nuclear medicine in that it uses a radiopharmaceutical agent injected into the circulatory system to image the area of interest. However, PET is also used to evaluate the physiologic condition or function of an organ or system in the body. The radiation emanates from the body and is received by radiation detectors. The resulting cross-sectional images indicate how the radiopharmaceutical agent was taken up and used by the body. Because this chemical is treated by the body much like its own naturally occurring components, the information acquired is a highly accurate representation of the function of the area in question.

Portable Radiography and Fluoroscopy

Portable radiography and fluoroscopy can be performed if the patient cannot be moved to the radiology department. Mobile radiography units operate with battery power. The quality of images of most anatomic structures is equivalent to that obtained in the radiology department. However, many radiographic procedures cannot be performed with a portable unit. Portable radiography is used in such areas as the surgical department or operating room (OR), postanesthesia care unit (PACU), intensive care unit (ICU), coronary care unit (CCU), neonatal intensive care unit (NICU), burn unit, orthopedic unit, and morgue.

Mobile fluoroscopy (C-arm) is used primarily in the OR, where the surgeon must see the images immediately. Portable fluoroscopy must be used with great care to prevent those involved—both workers and patients—from being unnecessarily irradiated.

Diagnostic Medical Sonography

Diagnostic medical sonography uses high-frequency sound waves, which is a form of nonionizing radiation, to obtain sectional images of the body. Originally used by the military to detect enemy submarines, sonography is a useful diagnostic tool in certain areas of radiology. The sound waves bounce off interior structures of the body and return as echoes to a probe from which images can be electronically displayed on a monitor; permanent images can then be made from the screen. Cross-sectional images of the body are obtained using this method. Evaluation of moving organs can also be made with sonography. A type of sonography known as the Doppler technique is used to evaluate blood flow through the arteries.

Picture Archiving and Communication System

After reading the descriptions of imaging equipment presented in this chapter, you can understand that computers play a vital role in radiologic technology. Computed imaging procedures such as DR, CT, nuclear medicine, digital sonography, and MRI can be combined into a network using a common language called **digital communications in medicine (DICOM)**. The **picture archiving and communication system (PACS)** brings digital imaging together with **hospital and radiology information systems (HIS, RIS)**; it allows for the total management of a patient's case.

PACS forms a network that can be accessed from any workstation that is connected to the system. Data are stored on servers. Information can be transmitted from the computer storage device via cable throughout the hospital and vicinity or via satellite across the world. Because the images are ultimately viewed on monitors, high-resolution monitors are of the utmost importance.

The ability to manage all imaging procedures—as well as examination, interpretations, scheduling, patient history, cost analyses, demographics, and billing—makes PACS an invaluable tool in total patient care (Figure 8.13)

CONCLUSION

Radiographic imaging is one of the most exciting activities in any hospital, but keeping abreast of the continual advances in imaging equipment is a challenge for all radiologic technologists. An in-depth knowledge of physics and equipment is a necessary basis for understanding the latest technologic advancements in radiography. Physics is not a topic to be feared; it should be seen as the basis for all of diagnostic imaging. In addition, the computer is a vital component of diagnostic imaging. Studying the operation and uses of computers in medicine is mandatory for anyone entering the field of radiography. With all of this knowledge and understanding, you will be prepared for the inevitable advances in imaging techniques and equipment.

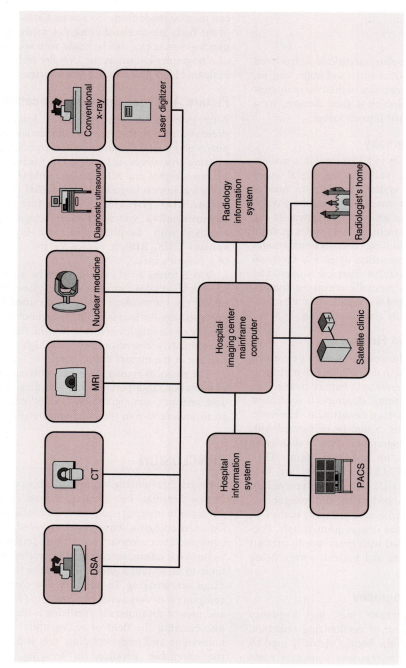

Fig. 8.13 The picture archiving and communication system (PACS) network integrates all imaging modalities, hospital information system and radiology information system, as well as local and remote workstations. *CT,* Computed tomography; *DSA,* digital subtraction angiography; *MRI,* magnetic resonance imaging. (From Bushong SC: *Radiologic science for technologists: physics, biology, and protection,* ed 11, St. Louis, 2017, Elsevier.)

QUESTIONS FOR DISCUSSION AND CRITICAL THINKING

1. Briefly describe the production of x-rays.
2. List the various densities in the human body as well as additional densities that may be encountered in imaging.
3. Compare kVp with mAs in their respective roles in x-ray production.
4. Describe the digital image properties of image brightness, contrast, and spatial resolution.
5. Explain how to manage the three types of image distortion.
6. Describe the required alignment of x-ray tube, anatomical part, and image receptor in creating a nondistorted image.
7. List examples of locations requiring the use of mobile radiography or mobile fluoroscopy.
8. Briefly describe the use of CT, MRI, sonography, and nuclear medicine.

BIBLIOGRAPHY

Bushong S. *Radiologic science for technologists.* ed 11. St. Louis: Elsevier; 2017.
Callaway W. *Mosby's comprehensive review of radiography.* ed 7. St. Louis: Elsevier; 2017.
Fauber T. Exposure variability and image quality in computed radiography. *Radiol Technol.* 2009; 80(3):209–215.
Fauber T. *Radiographic imaging and exposure.* ed 5. St. Louis: Elsevier; 2017.
Long B, Rollins J, Smith B. *Merrill's atlas of radiographic positioning and procedures.* ed 14. St. Louis: Elsevier; 2020.

9

Radiographic Examinations:
Diagnosing Disease and Injury

OBJECTIVES

On completion of this chapter, you should be able to:
- Describe internal and external patient preparation.
- Describe examinations that use iodine, barium, or air as a contrast agent.
- Describe what is included in skull and headwork radiography.
- Describe what is included in thoracic radiography.
- Describe what is included in extremity radiography.
- Describe what is included in spinal radiography.
- List conditions for which abdominal radiography may be performed.
- Briefly explain esophagograms, upper gastrointestinal series, small bowel studies, and barium enemas.
- List and describe the examinations that are referred to as *special imaging procedures*.

OUTLINE

Patient Preparation and Contrast Media
Radiographic Studies
   Skull and Headwork
   Thoracic Cavity
   Extremities
   Spine
   Abdomen
Fluoroscopic Examinations
   Esophagram
   Upper Gastrointestinal Series
   Barium Enema

   Urinary System Studies
   Endoscopic Retrograde Cholangiographic
      Pancreatography
Special Imaging Procedures
   Angiography and Interventional Procedures
   Arthrogram
   Hysterosalpingogram
   Mammogram
   Myelogram
Conclusion

KEY TERMS

angiogram
arthrogram
barium
barium enema
contrast media
cystogram

esophagram
excretory urography
external preparation
fluoroscopic studies
hysterosalpingogram
internal preparation

iodine
mammogram
myelogram
upper gastrointestinal series
voiding cystourethrogram

Radiography is one of the primary methods of diagnosing disease. Positioning and procedures will be covered in depth during your education, but this chapter provides an excellent overview of what you will observe and experience in the clinical setting. Not all institutions perform all of the procedures described here because hospital and clinic services vary. However, you should be familiar with all types of studies because your actual employment may be elsewhere. In addition, as a student radiographer, you must become competent in many of the procedures performed by diagnostic radiographers.

The radiographic examinations discussed in this chapter are divided into radiographic, fluoroscopic, and special imaging procedures. Bear in mind that some of these procedures may be performed using digital fluoroscopy, digital radiography, computed tomography (CT), or magnetic resonance imaging (MRI).

PATIENT PREPARATION AND CONTRAST MEDIA

Depending on the examination, patient preparation is performed either internally or externally. **External preparation** requires removing clothing and jewelry that may be covering the area of the body through which the x-rays must pass. Many types of clothing material show up on the image as obscure shadows. Buttons and zippers may hide small disease processes or fractures. If a region of the head is being radiographed, dentures must be removed because they interfere with the passage of x-rays through the mouth. Rings and watches must be removed when radiographing the hand or wrist. One of the most common mistakes is forgetting to remove a necklace before performing a chest examination (Fig. 9.1, *A*). Always ask each patient to remove jewelry before beginning an examination. In addition, ask the patient if the area of the body to be radiographed is pierced; if so, request that all piercing jewelry be removed from the body part. Failure to do so results in a double dose of radiation to the patient because the radiographs must be retaken. Note if a tattoo is in the area being radiographed. If the ink used in the tattoo contains metallic pigmentation, it may appear as a faint shadow on the radiographic image. Proper examination of the patient is the responsibility of the radiographer. Checks for unwanted objects should be verbal, visual, and tactile.

Internal preparation for some examinations includes cleansing enemas, which are performed so that structures in the abdomen are not obscured by gas and fecal material. Most of these preparations are administered on the nursing units or by the patient at home. However, awareness of hospital procedures helps explain the importance of this preparation and answers any questions the patient may have. As a competent radiographer, you must be aware of all aspects of patient care that relate to the examination, regardless of whether you perform them. Internal preparation may also include having the patient take nothing by mouth for several hours preceding the procedure.

Contrast media are solutions or gases introduced into the body to provide contrast on a radiograph between adjacent tissues. The three general types of contrast media used in radiography are (1) barium-based media, (2) iodine-based media, and (3) air.

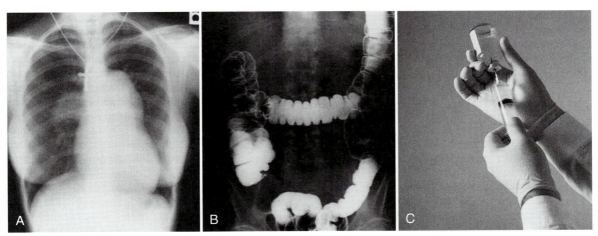

Fig. 9.1 A, Failure to remove a patient's jewelry results in the retaking of a radiograph. **B,** Contrast medium provides contrast between an organ and its surrounding tissue. **C,** Radiographer prepares an injection of an iodinated contrast agent.

The element **barium** has approximately the same contrast qualities as iodine, but the similarities end there. Barium sulfate is inert and cannot be absorbed by the body; this makes it the medium of choice for gastrointestinal (GI) studies (Fig. 9.1, *B*). Patient allergic reaction to barium is almost nonexistent because of its inert properties.

However, exceptions exist. For example, if surgery appears imminent or if a perforated stomach or intestine is suspected, barium would not be used because it cannot be absorbed. In such cases, a water-soluble iodine contrast agent is used because it is readily absorbed should spillage into the abdominal cavity occur.

The element **iodine** has a relatively high atomic number. Because x-rays do not readily pass through iodine, solutions that contain this element are placed in organs and blood vessels to provide a contrast between these structures and their surrounding tissues (Fig 9.1, *C*). The radiographer must be alert to possible adverse reactions the patient may experience when using iodinated contrast media. The use of nonionic contrast media greatly reduces the occurrence of such side effects, but it does not eliminate them.

Air is used as a contrast agent primarily in chest radiography. Unlike iodine and barium, air is easily penetrated by x-rays, thus providing contrast between lung tissue, vessel markings, and the air sacs themselves. Air may also be used with barium-based or iodine-based contrast media to provide a double contrast.

RADIOGRAPHIC STUDIES

Radiographic studies are examinations performed by the radiographer on particular regions of the body with the use of the x-ray tube. The images are acquired using digital imaging equipment and are subsequently interpreted by the radiologist. The radiographic examinations performed are listed in the following text according to body region, and a few comments are offered that will help you understand the studies.

Skull and Headwork

Radiographic studies of the region above the neck make up the skull and headwork category. Many of these procedures are performed primarily with CT or panoramic tomography. Examinations that may be performed include the skull, facial bones, nasal bones, mandible, temporomandibular joints (TMJs), and sinuses. These examinations require multiple views, and some can be rather difficult to perform. Headwork imaging is usually performed to evaluate possible fractures, locate foreign bodies, or examine abnormalities. Areas such as the sella turcica, zygomatic arches, mastoids, and orbits are primarily imaged using CT. The mandible and TMJs are normally using panoramic tomography.

Thoracic Cavity

The thoracic cavity includes the bones and tissues of the chest region and is the most commonly radiographed region of the body. Exact positioning and careful exposure techniques are essential for proper imaging. Other studies of the thoracic cavity include the ribs, sternoclavicular joints, and sternum. Thoracic studies may be performed to evaluate fluid in the lungs, overexpansion, collapsed lungs, tumors, heart enlargement, and other heart and lung abnormalities, as well as fractures of the ribs, sternoclavicular joints, and sternum.

Extremities

The extremities category is generally divided into the upper and lower regions and also includes the shoulder and pelvic regions. Upper extremity studies include radiographs of the fingers, hands, wrists, forearms, elbows, humeri, shoulders, clavicles, acromioclavicular joints, and scapulas. Lower extremity studies include radiographs of the toes, feet, heels, ankles, lower legs, knees, patellae, femurs, hips, and pelvis. Bone studies always require at least two views that are taken at right angles to one another; joint studies may also include an oblique view. Care must be taken when performing bone and joint studies because of the possibility of broken bones (fractures). Studies in patient care explain how injured patients are properly handled. Radiologic examinations of the extremities are performed to evaluate bone fractures, dislocations, arthritis, osteoporosis, and tumors.

Spine

The spine category includes studies of the cervical spine, thoracic (dorsal) spine, lumbar spine, sacroiliac joints, sacrum, and coccyx. In addition, examinations such as scoliosis evaluation and bone age determination are included in this category. Patients with spinal injuries must be carefully handled because further injury can result if the nerves are damaged. Spinal injuries are painful, and the radiographer must make the patient as comfortable as possible while obtaining as many diagnostic radiographs as necessary for the physician's evaluation. In addition to evaluating severe trauma, spinal studies are performed to evaluate the extent of arthritis of the spine, abnormal curvatures, muscle spasms that may be causing the spine to curve, and slipped vertebrae. Trauma studies of the cervical spine are primarily imaged with CT.

Abdomen

Many of the studies involving the abdomen require the use of fluoroscopy and are discussed more fully in the next section. However, some radiographic surveys are made of the abdomen without the use of contrast agents and fluoroscopy. Careful patient handling is important because many patients who are having abdomen examinations are quite ill and in pain. Again, providing proper care for the patient is your responsibility in the radiology department. Abdominal studies often determine the presence of foreign masses; calcifications; the distribution of air in the intestines; the size, shape, and location of major organs such as the liver, kidney, and spleen; and bony and soft-tissue damage. These studies are also used to evaluate individual organs, although most such studies are performed using CT.

FLUOROSCOPIC EXAMINATIONS

Fluoroscopic studies require a radiologist or radiologist assistant (RA) to perform and monitor the examination in most circumstances. Viewing the anatomy "live" or "dynamic" is necessary for proper diagnosis. The following discussion highlights the most commonly performed examinations. Images are acquired by the radiologist using digital fluoroscopy. Digital studies may involve postprocessing of the image by the radiologist.

Esophagram

The **esophagram**, which is a study of the esophagus, requires the patient to swallow a barium-sulfate preparation. The radiologist or RA obtains digital images. Often, the patient has difficulty swallowing the barium because of its thick, pastelike mixture that lingers in the esophagus. Esophagrams may visualize tumors, constrictions, and spasms.

Upper Gastrointestinal Series

Studies of the stomach, often called an **upper gastrointestinal series**, are performed with the use of barium sulfate. The patient must drink the solution while fluoroscopically controlled images are obtained. The upper GI series is performed to evaluate hiatal hernias, peptic ulcers, and other stomach disorders. If the small intestine must be evaluated, a small bowel examination is performed. This examination involves radiographing the abdomen every hour to watch the progress of the barium meal through the small intestine. Advising the patient ahead of time that this study will take several hours to perform is important. In certain cases, CT is also used as part of a small bowel examination. Small bowel studies are performed to investigate tumors, inflammation, obstructions, and the malabsorption of nutrients. Fiber-optic endoscopy is also used to examine the stomach.

Barium Enema

The radiographic examination of the colon, which is called a **barium enema**, involves introducing a barium solution into the colon. Although this study is not unduly painful, it is often considered uncomfortable. Because the barium solution may cause cramping and discomfort, the radiologist and radiographer must work rapidly and accurately so that the barium solution can be excreted as soon as possible. Glucagon is often used in air-contrast studies of the colon to reduce cramping and peristalsis. Barium studies may indicate tumors, bowel obstructions, diverticula, and inflammation. A study called the *air-contrast barium enema* is performed by introducing air in addition to the barium to provide a double contrast, which allows for better visualization of abnormalities in the colon such as diverticula and polyps.

Colonoscopy using an endoscope is proving to be a very effective tool in visualizing the colon. It also has the advantage of being able to obtain a biopsy at the same time. Both the colonoscopy and virtual colonoscopy, which is a CT procedure used to reconstruct the colon using computer images, play major roles in diagnosis.

Urinary System Studies

Examination of the urinary system is normally performed in tandem with CT. It may be performed as part of a study called **excretory urography**, which is also called *intravenous urography* or *intravenous pyelography* (IVP). Using CT, it is called a CT/IVP. When performed without CT, IVPs involve the use of an iodinated contrast agent injected into the bloodstream through a vein in the arm. Radiographs are obtained at intervals of several minutes during the time that the kidneys, ureters, and bladder are highlighted by the contrast material. Intravenous urography helps visualize stones in the urinary system and evaluate kidney function.

In addition to the IVPs, studies of the urinary system may be performed under fluoroscopic control. For example, the **cystogram**, which is a study of the urinary bladder, involves filling the bladder with a contrast agent and then taking radiographs of the bladder. A **voiding cystourethrogram**, which evaluates urination, is similar except that the patient empties the bladder while under fluoroscopic observation.

Endoscopic Retrograde Cholangiographic Pancreatography

An endoscopic retrograde cholangiographic pancreatography (ERCP) is performed to diagnose anomalies in the biliary system or pancreas. A contrast medium is injected into the common bile duct after it is located with an endoscope passed down the esophagus, through the stomach, and into the small intestine under fluoroscopic observation. Radiographic images may then be acquired.

SPECIAL IMAGING PROCEDURES

Certain imaging examinations require special equipment or are just not routinely performed. A brief description of the more common ones follows.

Angiography and Interventional Procedures

The **angiogram** is a study that visualizes the arteries of a particular body region. An iodine-based contrast material is injected, and a very rapid sequence of images is made. These images allow for the viewing of the blood flow through the artery and an evaluation of the shape and condition of the artery itself. Performing angiography involves the use of digital fluoroscopy, a ceiling mounted C-arm, automatic injector, and a sterile field (Fig. 9.2, *A*). These examinations are a part of interventional radiology, which may also involve angioplasty, a procedure that helps restore normal blood flow through the vessel. Imaging in angiography may also involve three-dimensional reconstruction of the images.

Arthrogram

Arthrography is normally performed in tandem with CT or MRI. Some physicians still prefer conventional arthrography. The **arthrogram** is used to evaluate the structures in and around a joint space. The most common joints involved are the knee and shoulder. An iodinated contrast medium is injected directly into the joint space. Fluoroscopy is used and images are obtained by the radiologist.

Hysterosalpingogram

The **hysterosalpingogram** is an examination of the uterus and fallopian tubes. This examination allows for the evaluation of the shape of the uterus and patency of the oviducts. An oil-based iodinated contrast medium is used to fill these structures. Fluoroscopy is used, and follow-up images may also be obtained.

Mammogram

A **mammogram** is a radiographic study of the breast. Because breast tissue has little inherent contrast, high-contrast imaging is required for proper diagnosis. The breast is compressed to allow for maximum visualization. Modern imaging equipment provides the detail that is of critical importance in the early detection of breast cancer. Breast imaging rooms include digital mammography units many of which are capable of 3D image production.

Myelogram

The **myelogram** is an examination of the subarachnoid space of the spinal cord (Fig. 9.2, *B*). After the removal of some of the spinal fluid, a water-soluble iodine-contrast agent is injected into the space through the patient's back or neck. Fluoroscopy is used to guide the flow of the contrast agent and to obtain images of the region. The patient may be given a sedative, which causes drowsiness; therefore patient care must be at its best. Myelography is often used in tandem with CT or MRI.

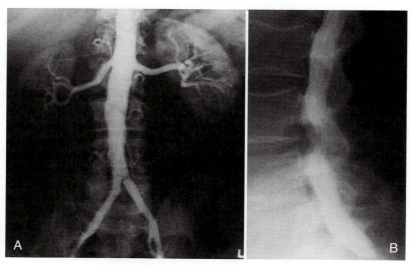

Fig. 9.2 A, Arteriogram. **B,** Myelogram.

CONCLUSION

The preceding discussion of radiographic, fluoroscopic, and special imaging examinations is not meant to be all-inclusive; the studies described in this text are the ones that you will most likely see in average and large departments. Smaller departments may never perform some of the procedures; others are involved with even more specialized studies. The step-by-step procedures for performing these examinations will be presented in your course on radiographic procedures. However, you may soon be observing these procedures or hearing discussions about them. This basic knowledge of examinations will help you become oriented to the clinical environment.

QUESTIONS FOR DISCUSSION AND CRITICAL THINKING

1. Discuss the importance of external and internal patient preparation, including its role in radiation protection.
2. Compare the use of barium and iodine in contrast examinations.
3. Discuss the primary advantage of using fluoroscopy.
4. Describe the increasing role of computed tomography and magnetic resonance imaging in radiographic examinations.

BIBLIOGRAPHY

Callaway W. *Mosby's comprehensive review of radiography,* ed 7. St. Louis: Elsevier; 2017.

Long B, Rollins J, Smith B. *Merrill's atlas of radiographic positioning and procedures.* ed 14. St. Louis: Elsevier; 2020.

10

Radiation Safety and Protective Measures

OBJECTIVES

On completion of this chapter, you should be able to:

- Explain the need for radiation protection efforts by operators of radiation-producing equipment.
- List sources of radiation and explain their significance in dose accumulation.
- Define SI units of radiation measurement.
- Describe the role of the National Council on Radiation Protection and Measurements.
- Explain what is meant by as low as reasonably achievable (ALARA) for radiation workers.

- List and explain the two types of radiation–matter interactions that are significant in radiography.
- List and explain the four possible results that may occur when photons of radiation strike cells.
- List and explain the significance of radiation effects on the total body.
- List and describe the practical radiation protection methods expected of all radiologic technologists.
- Name two devices for monitoring personnel exposure to radiation.

OUTLINE

Need for Radiation Protection
    National Council on Radiation Protection and Measurements
    Radiation Measurements
Interaction of X-Rays With Matter
    Photoelectric Effect
    Compton Scatter
Biologic Effects of Ionizing Radiation
    Acute Radiation Syndrome
    Long-Term Effects
Sources of Exposure

    X-Rays
    Radionuclides
Primary Principles of Radiation Protection
Patient Protection
    Exposure Factors
    Collimation
    Repeat Exposures
    Gonadal Shielding
Personnel Protection
    Personnel Monitoring
Conclusion

KEY TERMS

air kerma
as low as reasonably achievable
background radiation
Becquerel (Bq)
carcinogenic
collimation
Compton scatter

deoxyribonucleic acid (DNA)
dosimetry
effective dose limit
erythema dose
gonad
gray (Gy)
human-made radiation

ionizing radiation
inverse square law
latent period
lymphocytes
photoelectric effect
sievert (Sv)

The well-known fact is that **ionizing radiation**, which is radiation that has sufficient energy to produce ions (e.g., x-rays), causes damage to living cells—damage that may be repaired, that may be permanent, or that may cause death to the cell. Therefore, everyone involved in the medical application of ionizing radiation must have a basic knowledge of the many ways to minimize its lethal and sublethal effects.

NEED FOR RADIATION PROTECTION

The two sources of ionizing radiation to which everyone is exposed are (1) natural environmental or background radiation and (2) human-made radiation. Examples of natural environmental or **background radiation** include cosmic radiation from the sun and stars; radioactive elements in the earth, such as uranium, radium, and thorium; and other radioactive substances that are found in foods, drinking water, and the air. Most of our exposure to natural background radiation comes from radon gas.

The amount of radiation that we receive from our natural environment depends to a great extent on where we live. One area of India has a high intensity of background radioactivity that gives the population 10 times more radiation than the average background radiation dose in the United States. People who live in high-altitude areas receive more cosmic radiation than those living in low-altitude areas; for example, the population in and around mile-high Denver receives more radiation than populations in or near sea-level coastal areas. Although background radiation varies from place to place, it accounts for more than one half of the exposure that the general public receives. Radiation has existed since time began. Diseases resulting from excessive radiation are not new, either. The same kinds of harmful effects that radiation causes can also be caused by other agents, such as certain chemicals.

Human-made radiation sources include (1) fallout from nuclear weapons testing and effluents from nuclear power plants, (2) radioactive materials used in industry, and (3) medical and dental x-ray exposures. The use of medical and dental radiographs and radioactive materials to diagnose and treat disease accounts for most of general public's exposure to human-made radiation.

The possibility of radiation-induced injury was reported shortly after Roentgen's discovery of x-rays in 1895. Since then, research, advanced technology, and the communications media have made society increasingly aware of the possible harmful effects of radiation; this awareness has led to a belief that patient exposure to ionizing radiation must be kept to a minimum while obtaining optimal diagnostic information for the radiologist. Understanding the characteristics of x-radiation, its biologic effects, and the methods of reducing patient and operator exposure is the responsibility of the radiologic technologist.

National Council on Radiation Protection and Measurements

In 1964, the Congress of the United States chartered the National Council on Radiation Protection and Measurements (NCRP) as a nonprofit corporation. The NCRP is composed of scientific committees the members of which are experts in their particular field or area of interest, and its primary function is to provide information and recommendations in the public interest about radiation measurements and protection. Another of its functions is to allow a pooling of resources from organizations to facilitate studies in radiation measurements and protection. A third function is to develop basic concepts about radiation protection and measurements and to develop the applications of these concepts. Last, the council makes a concerted effort to cooperate with international governmental and private organizations with regard to radiation measurements and protection.

Nuclear power production and the use of certain radioactive materials generally come under the control of the Atomic Energy Commission. Environmental radiologic health protection is usually the responsibility of the Environmental Protection Agency.

Radiation Measurements

As awareness of the possible dangers of x-ray use increased, establishing a method of measuring its use became necessary. In the early days, persons who worked with x-rays used a unit of measure called the **erythema dose**. This unit was the amount of radiation required to turn the skin red, and its name was derived from the term *erythema*, which means redness of the skin. However, the erythema dose lacked preciseness and accuracy.

Units of measurement of radiation have evolved to the current use of the International System of Units (SI). In general, those units are **air kerma**, for measuring radiation dose in air, **gray (Gy)** for absorbed dose, and **sievert (Sv)** for effective dose. The unit of activity is the **Becquerel (Bq)**; this measure is used in nuclear medicine studies with radionuclides. Table 10.1 shows the specific use of each unit of measurement.

Effective Dose Limits

The term **effective dose limit** is in adherence to the radiation protection guides. The philosophy underlying the establishment of dose limits is twofold: The first premise is the nonthreshold concept, and the second is the risks-versus-benefits relationship. Simply stated, the nonthreshold concept is the belief that no known level of radiation exposure exists below which adverse biologic effects may

TABLE 10.1   Units of Measurement

Measurement	Unit of Measurement	Symbol
Air kerma: unit of exposure	Gray, in air	Gy_a
Absorbed dose, energy absorbed per unit mass of tissue	Gray, in tissue	Gy_t
Equivalent dose or dose equivalent	Sievert	Sv
Effective dose	Sievert	Sv
Activity	Becquerel	Bq

TABLE 10.2   Effective Dose Limits (Annual)

Area Affected	Limit (mSv)
Occupational worker: whole body	50
Occupational worker: cumulative	10 mSv × age (years)
Occupational worker: lens of the eye	150
Occupational worker: localized areas of the skin, hands, and feet	500
General public, frequent exposure	1
General public, infrequent exposure	5
Embryo or fetus, per month during gestation	0.5
Embryo or fetus, total for gestation	5

not occur. This theory is backed primarily by the observation of clinically induced irradiation to animals and extrapolation of high-dose irradiation received by atomic bomb survivors. If the assumption is that any amount of radiation can possibly cause deleterious effects to humans, then all radiation must be used prudently for the benefit of all concerned. The phrase, **as low as reasonably achievable** (ALARA), is the basis for the NCRP establishment of policies and procedures for radiation exposure.

The primary goal of radiation protection of the individual is to keep exposure to a level below which adverse effects may be apparent during the lifespan as well as to keep exposure to the population gene pool as low as reasonable. Whenever physicians order a radiographic procedure, they must weigh the benefits to be obtained against the risk of the exposure. Although every effort should be exerted to keep the dose of radiation at the lowest possible level for people who are well, this effort should not be a deterrent for the use of x-radiation for the detection and identification of disease processes in patients who are injured or ill, provided this use is performed by physicians and radiologic technologists who are trained and experienced in making such examinations.

Dose limits are categorized into two groups: radiation workers and the general public. Table 10.2 summarizes the dose limits. Regarding the embryo or fetal dose, it is advisable, if possible, to postpone *all* radiation exposure during the entire gestation period or to use another imaging modality, such as sonography, to gather information for diagnosis (Fig. 10.1).

The nonthreshold concept and risks-versus-benefits relationship should always be kept in mind when considering the use of ionizing radiation in patient diagnoses. The information gained from a diagnostic radiograph should be far more beneficial than the possible risks incurred by exposure of the patient to ionizing radiation.

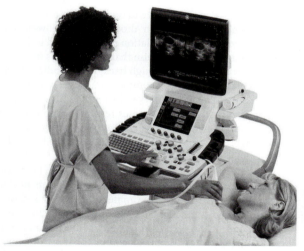

Fig. 10.1 Sonography is often used to obtain diagnostic information on pregnant women. X-radiation can be dangerous to a developing embryo or fetus. (From Lampignano J, Kendrick L: *Bontrager's textbook of radiographic positioning and related anatomy*, ed 9, St. Louis, 2018, Elsevier.)

INTERACTION OF X-RAYS WITH MATTER

An atom is the smallest part of an element and is made up of a nucleus surrounded by electrons. X-rays are packets of energy called photons, which have the ability to knock electrons out of their orbit; this action creates electrically charged ions. When x-rays pass through matter (tissue), this process of ionization results in a transfer of energy. The x-ray photons can be absorbed or scattered by the medium with which the photons interact or pass directly through the medium without any interaction taking place. The two main types of photon interactions that are important to diagnostic radiography are photoelectric effect and Compton interaction.

Photoelectric Effect

Photoelectric effect (Fig. 10.2, *A*) is the most common process of energy transfer that occurs when ionizing radiation interacts with matter. The process begins when a photon (a packet of energy) knocks an inner-orbit electron out of orbit and transfers all of its energy to the electron. The photon then no longer exists, and the electron becomes a photoelectron that possesses sufficient energy to knock electrons of other atoms from their orbit. The photoelectron and the atom from which it left are known as an *ion pair*. Photoelectric effect usually occurs with low-energy photons. The photoelectron may have sufficient energy to cause further ionizing reactions.

Compton Scatter

Compton scatter (Figs. 10.2, *B* and 10.3) is characterized by an incoming photon interacting with an orbital electron. In this case, only a portion of the incident photon's energy is transferred to the orbital electron; the orbital electron is then known as the *ejected Compton electron,* and it produces secondary ionization in the same manner as the photoelectron. The incident photon then becomes a scattered photon of lower energy, and it moves in a different direction and is capable of interacting with other atoms by Compton or photoelectric effect. The energy of the scattered photon is dependent on the energy of the incident photon and the angle between the incident and scattered photon. A type of scattering exists in which the entering photon changes direction but does not give up any of its energy; this type is called *unmodified, coherent,* or *classic scattering.* When a collision occurs and the photon gives up part of its energy in removing an electron, it is called *modified scattering.*

BIOLOGIC EFFECTS OF IONIZING RADIATION

The cell is a highly organized structure that is composed of a nucleus that is surrounded by cytoplasm. The cytoplasm contains structures that are responsible for protein synthesis and metabolism that is essential to normal body functions. The nucleus contains chromosomes, and these chromosomes contain genes. Genes are molecules that

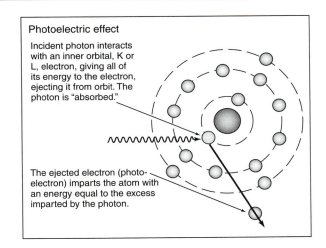

Photoelectric effect

Incident photon interacts with an inner orbital, K or L, electron, giving all of its energy to the electron, ejecting it from orbit. The photon is "absorbed."

The ejected electron (photoelectron) imparts the atom with an energy equal to the excess imparted by the photon.

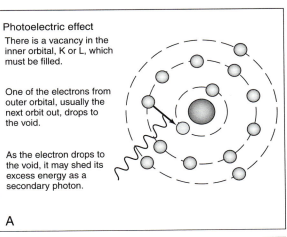

Photoelectric effect

There is a vacancy in the inner orbital, K or L, which must be filled.

One of the electrons from outer orbital, usually the next orbit out, drops to the void.

As the electron drops to the void, it may shed its excess energy as a secondary photon.

A

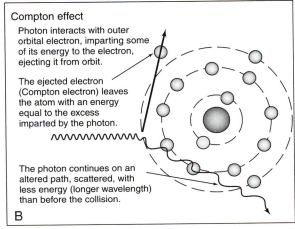

Compton effect

Photon interacts with outer orbital electron, imparting some of its energy to the electron, ejecting it from orbit.

The ejected electron (Compton electron) leaves the atom with an energy equal to the excess imparted by the photon.

The photon continues on an altered path, scattered, with less energy (longer wavelength) than before the collision.

B

Fig. 10.2 A, Photoelectric x-ray interaction with matter. **B,** Compton x-ray interaction with matter.

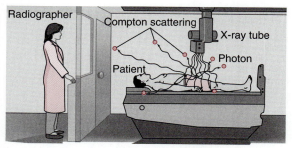

Fig. 10.3 Compton interaction produces scatter radiation in multiple directions. Compton interaction may expose an unshielded radiographer. (From Statkiewicz Sherer MA, Visconti PJ, et al: *Radiation protection in medical radiography*, ed 8, St. Louis, 2018, Elsevier.)

contain the genetic material that is responsible for transmitting hereditary information and controlling cytoplasmic activities. The genetic material is called **deoxyribonucleic acid (DNA)**, and it is described as a double-helix structure. This structure is best pictured as a flexible rope ladder that is twisted in a spiral staircase shape. All parts of the cell have an equal chance to be affected by ionization. Because the DNA molecule is less than 1% of the cell, DNA is hit less frequently than water molecules. However, damage to the DNA is more critical than damage to the water molecules.

The two basic types of cells are (1) germ cells, which are responsible for sexual reproduction, and (2) somatic cells, which perform all other body functions. Germ cells contain 23 chromosomes, and they are able to function with one half of the normal number of 46 chromosomes because of their specialization. Somatic cells must carry on many different functions and cannot survive or function normally without maintaining 46 chromosomes.

When radiation hits a cell, four possible results occur:
1. The radiation may pass through the cell without doing any damage.
2. It may temporarily damage the cell, but the cell subsequently regains normal functions.
3. It may damage the cell and no repair takes place.
4. It may kill the cell.

One theory about radiation exposure to the cell is known as the direct-hit theory. This theory asserts that when ionizing radiation interacts directly with the DNA molecule, certain breaks can occur in the "rung" of the DNA "ladder." If two direct hits occur to the same rung of the ladder, then a section of the chromosome is deleted. When the division process of mitosis occurs, incorrect amounts of genetic material are given to the new daughter cells. Mitosis is the process of somatic cell division whereby a parent cell divides to make two daughter cells that are replicas of the parent. These new cells either die or function abnormally because of the incorrect amount of genetic material in each cell.

The indirect theory involves radiation reacting with water in the cell. Various ions and free radicals form and may react with the cell or recombine to form a cellular poison. In this instance, the cell may be damaged or indirectly destroyed, but it is injured nonetheless.

As cells differ in their functions, they also differ in their rates of division or mitotic rate. Bergonie and Tribondeau established a law about the sensitivity of cells to ionizing radiation. The law of Bergonie and Tribondeau states:

Cells are most sensitive to the effects of ionizing radiation when they are immature, undifferentiated, and rapidly dividing.

Some specific cells that can be categorized by Bergonie and Tribondeau's law are mature white blood cells called **lymphocytes**. These cells are considered the most radiosensitive cells. Cells that make up the lens of the eye, the ovaries, and the testes are also known to be extremely radiosensitive. Cells that make up skin tissue and that line other body organs such as the bladder, the esophagus, and the rectum are moderately sensitive. Nerve cells are the least sensitive because they are highly differentiated and do not divide; these cells are said to be radioresistant.

Fortunately, irradiated cells that have been damaged are capable of repair; however, in some instances, complete repair is not possible, and cells are often incorrectly repaired. Over time, incomplete or incorrect repair is responsible for the development of adverse effects to the body. The term **latent period** is the time between the initial irradiation and the occurrence of any biologic change. The response of a cell to radiation exposure depends on the radiosensitivity of the cell, the type of radiation (alpha, gamma, x-ray), the rate of radiation, and the total dose level.

Acute Radiation Syndrome

Biologic effects of ionizing radiation that appear in minutes, hours, days, or weeks are known as short-term effects. The signs and symptoms that comprise these short-term effects are the acute radiation syndrome (ARS) that occurs when a very large dose is received by the entire body over a short time period. The important points to remember about acute radiation syndrome are that it is a total-body response to a large dose received over a short time period and that it is characterized by short-term biologic effects. Irradiating a smaller body area with a similar large dose is possible, but this would produce less critical biologic effects than those exhibited by a total-body response. ARS is not possible at diagnostic doses of x-radiation.

Long-Term Effects

Long-term biologic effects of ionizing radiation are divided into two categories: (1) somatic effects and (2) genetic effects. Somatic effects occur in general body cells that involve all body functions except sexual reproduction. These effects include cancer, cataracts, and life-span shortening. Long-term effects may not become apparent for periods of 1 to 30 years and therefore are difficult to assess as being specifically radiation induced. These effects in individuals may be the result of a previous acute high-dose exposure or of chronic low-dose radiation exposures.

Somatic Effects

Birth defects are considered a possible long-term effect of the irradiation of the embryo of a pregnant woman. Some defects exhibited at birth may be genetic in nature. Genetic defects are a result of prior damage to the gene cells that participate in the formation of an embryo. Genetic material may be damaged by agents other than radiation, but radiation-induced damage is the concern here. Defects induced by radiation in the organism may occur at the genetic, embryonic, or fetal stage. Such effects exhibit as forms of mental retardation and skeletal and central nervous system abnormalities. Irradiated embryos also tend to develop childhood leukemia in a greater proportion than do nonirradiated embryos, but the possibility of any effect from diagnostic doses is extremely remote. Because its cells are dividing so rapidly and are still undifferentiated at this stage, an embryo is particularly sensitive to the adverse effects of radiation at extremely low doses, per the law of Bergonie and Tribondeau.

Radiation has long been accepted as a **carcinogenic** (cancer-causing) agent. Early evidence of its carcinogenic effects was seen in an increase in bone sarcomas of radium dial painters. Paint containing small amounts of radium was ingested by these individuals when they pointed the tips of their brushes with their lips or tongues while painting the luminous dials on watches. Many early radiologists and technicians also exhibited skin carcinomas from occupational exposures. Lung cancer resulting from the inhalation of radioactive materials in the air was present in many uranium mineworkers. Other types of cancers can also be radiation induced.

Evidence of radiation-induced cataracts came from heavily irradiated atomic bomb survivors, a small number of workers accidentally exposed to very high doses, and several nuclear physicists who were working with cyclotrons. The general consensus is that the eye lens is extremely radiosensitive.

The first indication of a decreased life span was observed in studies of American radiologists compared with other physicians. Because of the many variables involved with this long-term effect, much controversy continues over the assumption that radiation induces a shortened life span; it is, however, based on the apparent fact of a smaller differential in each new life-span comparison. This trend tends to reinforce the assumption that early radiologists were exposed to larger amounts of radiation because of the lack of safety precautions and more primitive technology, which created a life span–shortening effect.

Long-term epidemiological studies have been performed on radiologic technologists. No shortening of life span has been shown to be caused by working in radiology.

Genetic Effects

Genetic effects are the second category associated with the long-term biologic effects of ionizing radiation. Genetic effects occur in the germ cells, which are responsible for sexual reproduction. The effects that occur within the germ cell are transmitted to future generations and are therefore not evident to the individual in which they initially take place. To transmit genetic information, DNA sends messages in codes. When any part of this code sequence is broken, an incorrect message is transmitted. Any alteration in the structure or amount of DNA is called a *mutation*. When radiation damages a chromosome of a male sperm or a female egg, the possibility of transmitting a mutation or distorted genetic information to future generations occurs.

Remember that germ cells genes contain 23 separate chromosomes and that when a female germ cell unites with a male germ cell, they form a cell (called a *zygote*) that contains 46 chromosomes. When a genetic mutation develops in a chromosome, it is usually recessive and does not have a correct message to transmit. However, if one recessive gene is found in the sperm and the same recessive gene is present in the ovum, the genetic mutation will express itself in the resulting zygote or mature offspring.

Considerations when assessing the possibility of radiation-induced genetic mutations include the following:

1. Other agents that can cause possible gene mutations are drugs, increased body temperature, chemicals, and viruses.
2. A certain number of spontaneous mutations occur in every generation.
3. The gonads of the individual may have been exposed to ionizing radiation.
4. Mutations may not occur in successive generations because of limited life span, small number of offspring, and the unlikelihood of two recessive genes.
5. No threshold apparently exists below which no genetic mutations occur.

6. The increase in society's mobility, number of marriages per person, and crossing of socioeconomic backgrounds increases the probability of recessive genes manifesting themselves in future generations.
7. Radiation-induced mutations cannot be distinguished from mutations caused by other mutagens.
8. Mutations are irreversible and inherited.

Ways in which genetic mutations can become apparent are miscarriages, physical birth defects, and metabolic or biologic changes causing a predisposition to disease or premature death.

Numerous factors that influence the biologic effects of ionizing radiation on cells, tissues, and organs of humans have been covered. Students should remember that some of the biologic effects are theories established from early unprotected use of radiation and laboratory findings in animals; radiation-induced genetic damage is one such theory that was introduced.

SOURCES OF EXPOSURE

The two sources of medical radiation exposure are x-rays and radionuclides. X-rays are considered an external source, and radionuclides are an internal source.

X-Rays

X-rays are produced whenever a stream of high-speed electrons hits the atoms of a metal target in an x-ray tube. A high voltage (also called *kilovoltage*) must be applied to the tube to accelerate the electrons; the kilovoltage controls the quality of the x-ray beam. *Milliamperage* (mA) controls the quantity or amount of radiation produced and functions inside the tube. The resulting x-rays are emitted through a port that is often called a window. The radiographic tube is usually housed above the x-ray table and, except for a portable x-ray machine, is normally suspended from the ceiling on a movable track. The x-rays produced from this tube are called *primary* radiation. Easily absorbed, harmful soft x-rays are removed by a filter placed in the port of the x-ray tube housing. When this primary radiation interacts with matter, such as the patient, table, or image receptor, it results in two other types of radiation: (1) secondary radiation and (2) scattered radiation. Scattered radiation is not only harmful to the patient, but it also impairs the diagnostic quality of the image.

Additionally, another radiographic tube, called the *fluoroscopic x-ray tube,* may be inside the radiographic table. Generally, this tube is operated by the radiologist, and it allows for the viewing of an immediate image of the patient or body part. Primary, secondary, and scatter radiations are also emitted from this tube. X-ray tubes produce an external source of radiation.

Radionuclides

An internal source of radiation is produced by radionuclides, which are injected into the body tagged to radiopharmaceuticals. This source of radiation is used in the field of nuclear medicine. It is also used in the treatment of patients with cancer in radiation therapy. As radionuclides disintegrate, they emit gamma radiation, which is similar to x-rays but more penetrating. The value and effectiveness of a radionuclide is related to its half-life. The radioactive half-life of a substance is the time required for the activity of that nuclide to be reduced to one half of its initial value. More simply, half-life is the time needed for the disintegration of one half of the atoms of the nuclide.

PRIMARY PRINCIPLES OF RADIATION PROTECTION

The methods of protection from external radiation are time, distance, and shielding. The shorter the time period a person is exposed to radiation, the lower the dose will be. Shielding is an attempt to stop radiation in its path; shielding material absorbs the energy of the x-ray beam. The most effective protection from x-ray exposure is distance. The greater the distance between the source of radiation and the individual, the lower the dose will be.

PATIENT PROTECTION

Learning the philosophy, factors, and methods that minimize ionizing radiation exposure to the patient is the responsibility of the radiologic technologist. Even more essential is the adoption of this responsibility into the everyday work habits and decision-making processes. Estimates indicate that 65% of the population of the United States receives an x-ray examination each year. A significantly lower total population dose could be received by Americans if all radiologic technologists would use patient protection methods.

Again, the philosophy that governs radiation protection and safety is the nonthreshold concept. The acceptance of this approach should minimize the possibility of creating deleterious radiation effects.

Exposure Factors

The exposure factors of kilovoltage (kVp), milliampereseconds (mAs), and distance are directly related to the amount of radiation exposure a patient receives. Optimal (as high as possible) kilovoltage should be used unless it interferes with the study or diagnosis. The result is a decreased skin dose because of a decrease in the number of photoelectric interactions with tissue. The lowest possible mAs should be used to decrease patient dose and reduce the chance of motion unless a breathing technique with longer time is warranted for radiographs of the ribs, thoracic spine, or sternum. In fluoroscopy, the length of exposure to the patient is the key in determining the patient's total dose.

The rate of exposure is directly related to distance as a function of the **inverse square law**. The farther patients are from a source of radiation, the less exposure they will receive. With this fact in mind, the inverse square law states the following: the intensity of the beam is inversely proportional to the square of the distance.

In other words, as the distance between the patient and the x-ray tube increases, the exposure rate (intensity) decreases. Therefore, optimal x-ray tube (source) to image receptor distance (SID) must always be used.

Filtration

Filtration is another factor that affects patient exposure. In diagnostic radiology, aluminum is usually the metal used to absorb the harmful soft radiation. Radiographic tubes are manufactured with an inherent filtration of 0.5- to 0.9-mm aluminum or its equivalent. The minimal total filtration of the primary x-ray beam must be at least 2.5-mm aluminum or its equivalent when above 70 kVp. The absorption increases as filtration is added and kVp is decreased.

Grids

Grids are used to absorb the scattered radiation that is created by the interaction of primary radiation with matter before this scatter reaches the image receptor. Several types of grids are available, but they all use radiation-absorbing material to remove scattered radiation that would otherwise reach the image receptor and reduce diagnostic quality. Grid use, however, raises the patient dose. As digital imaging evolves, in some cases, software is able to remove the effects of scatter from the digital signal, thus eliminating the need for using grids.

Collimation

Collimation is the restriction of the primary radiation to a limited area. For example, if the primary beam is allowed to leave the tube port, it may cover an area that measures 20 cm × 25 cm. If the beam is restricted by the use of collimators, the area covered might be 17 cm × 20 cm. Collimators are located on the tube housing and can be manually adjusted to allow the x-radiation to cover an area smaller than the desired size.

Positive beam limitation (PBL) automatically adjusts the exposure area to the size of the image receptor; in most instances, the radiographer has the option to decrease the area covered even more. Using one-size image receptors

does require the radiographer to use collimation to restrict the beam to the specific area of interest in the patient.

Repeat Exposures

Repeat exposures double the dose to the patient for each projection repeated. They should be avoided as much as possible. Using optimal radiographic technique for the patient and pathology can greatly reduce repeats and subsequent radiation dose to the patient.

Gonadal Shielding

Gonad shields are available to protect reproductive cells. A **gonad** is the general term that describes both the male and female reproductive organs. Gonad shields should be used whenever the reproductive organs are in the primary beam if the area shielded is not necessary for the diagnosis (Fig. 10.4). Research has demonstrated that a 95% exposure reduction is possible when the testes have been shielded; ovaries can be protected up to a 50% reduction in exposure. Because of the location of the ovaries, they are more difficult to shield without compromising the diagnosis.

The usual gonadal shield is a flat contact shield made of lead-impregnated material. It may be a lead strip or a lead apron. Because positioning of the contact shield over the gonads by the technologist creates the possibility of embarrassment to both parties, experts suggest that the radiographer explain to the patient the shield's placement and its function.

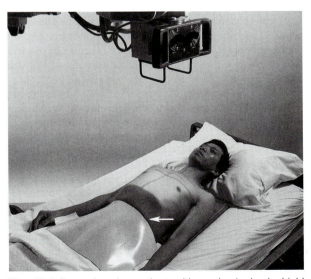

Fig. 10.4 Protecting the patient with a simple lead shield reduces exposure to parts of the body that are not imaged. (From Long B, Rollins J, Smith B: *Merrill's atlas of radiographic positioning and procedures*, ed 14, St. Louis, 2020, Elsevier.)

Examinations that give the patient a high-exposure dose to the gonads are the hip, upper femur, lumbar spine, sacrum, coccyx, sacroiliac joints, barium enema, and urography examinations.

Patient exposure can be reduced tremendously when the radiographer uses gonadal shielding. The technologist must take the time and effort to use shielding as an effective means of reducing genetic risks for the whole population.

PERSONNEL PROTECTION

Radiologic technologists who receive chronic low doses of radiation are more likely to be affected by its harmful effects if protective measures are not used. The factors and methods discussed for minimizing patient exposure are equally effective for reducing personnel exposure.

Researchers have proven distance can be employed to reduce the amount of exposure a technologist receives. This is of particular importance when the technologist is assisting with fluoroscopic procedures or operating a portable x-ray unit. The same inverse square law that protects patients also can be used to protect the technologist. It can be summarized in this way: when the distance from the source of radiation is doubled, the intensity of the radiation will be four times lower (one-fourth the exposure rate). This is a substantial reduction in radiation dose to the radiographer. Conversely, when the distance between the radiographer and the source of radiation is cut in half, the resulting exposure rate is increased four times.

During fluoroscopy, stand back from the x-ray table several feet unless you must attend to the patient or assist the radiologist. When performing portable radiography, use the exposure cord all the way out to its distance of 6 feet. Although these two practices reduce your dose, it is also critical to wear a lead apron (Box 10.1).

The safest place for the operator to stand during any radiographic exposure is in a shielded booth. If unavailable, a portable shield should be used to ensure protection. Just as other shielding devices are, the portable shield is lined with lead. Radiologic technologists should remember to keep their entire bodies within the shielded area, or they have negated its function. Loud, distinct communication and visual contact with the patient can be maintained through the shield's window. In most instances, the radiographic unit located within a shielded booth has a short exposure cord or a control panel exposure switch to inhibit the technologist from leaning outside the booth's protective confines.

Radiologic technologists should not hold patients or image receptors for an exposure. There are sufficient devices available to help with both, including tape, sandbags, wood blocks, and radiopaque sponges as well as image receptor holders.

BOX 10.1   Practical Applications to Keep the Technologist's Dose Low

Source of radiographer exposure: Compton interaction from the patient

Occurrence: fluoroscopy and portable radiography

Protection: lead apron. Always wear a lead apron when in fluoroscopy (including C-arm in surgery) and when performing portable radiography (use of the 6-ft exposure switch cord is important but does not shield the radiographer; scatter radiation still reaches the radiographer).

Protection: inverse square Law. Increase the distance from the source of radiation. Doubling the distance from the patient reduces radiographer dose to ¼, or four times lower than standing next to the patient. That is a substantial reduction in radiation dose to the radiographer.

Fluoroscopy: Stand back from the x-ray table several feet unless you must attend to the patient or assist the radiologist.

Portable radiography: It is critical to wear a lead apron. Use the exposure cord all the way out to its distance of 6 feet. If you are not the one making the exposure, step back even farther.

Keep in mind, the closer you are to the Compton scatter exiting the patient, your dose increases quickly. If the distance between the radiographer and the source of radiation is cut in half, the resulting exposure to the radiographer goes up four times.

If, after all techniques and solutions have been exhausted, a patient must be held, certain conditions must be met. First, the person restraining the patient should wear a lead apron, gloves, and protective glasses. A monitoring device should be worn by all radiologic technologists. If a layperson will be holding the patient and does not have a monitoring device, record the date, time, technique, and number of exposures. The restraining individual MUST stand out of the primary beam of radiation to minimize the radiation exposure received. At no time must anyone assisting be struck by the primary x-ray beam.

Personnel Monitoring

Although many radiation exposure monitoring devices are available, the optically stimulated luminescent dosimeter (OSL) and thermoluminescent dosimeter (TLD) are the ones used most often. The radiologic technologist should wear the dosimeter at all times during working hours. The dosimeter should be worn near the neck so that the exposure reading will closely represent the dose received by the eyes

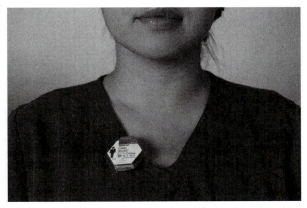

Fig. 10.5 A personal dosimeter worn at collar level outside of the lead apron. (From Lampignano J, Kendrick L: *Bontrager's textbook of radiographic positioning and related anatomy*, ed 9, St. Louis, 2018, Elsevier.)

and the thyroid. The radiologic technologist must wear the dosimeter in a consistent location (Fig. 10.5).

Generally, the dosimeter is removed and changed monthly or quarterly. A responsible and knowledgeable individual such as a health physicist or radiation safety officer should interpret and record monthly exposure records for each radiologic technologist. Accuracy in interpretation and recording are necessary because this information becomes a permanent part of the employee's record. Employers are required to maintain exposure dose records that are made available to employees and new employers.

In most cases, radiographers and students will be required to initial the dosimeter report indicating they have read it and understand their dose. This field of radiation monitoring is called **dosimetry**.

CONCLUSION

Radiation safety measures are essential in radiography for the protection of the patient, the radiographer, and others who may receive radiation during the course of their duties. Reasonable and achievable safe limits of radiation exposure must be established and practiced. Standards that shape the rules and regulations for radiation protection are based on experience, observations, and scientific research regarding radiation exposure and its effects on living tissue.

Students who aspire to become radiologic technologists should become familiar with the rules, regulations, opportunities, and philosophies that allow them to deliver optimal radiologic health care to patients with a minimum of radiation exposure. The radiation safety officer or radiation protection supervisor is responsible for monitoring exposure rates, designating radiation areas with proper warning signs, and ensuring that equipment monitoring and safety checks are made. Continued research for increased radiation protection and safety measures affords radiologic technologists the opportunity to become aware of innovative methods, ideas, and products in this area.

It is up to the radiographer to use distance and lead shielding as effective means of reducing their own radiation dose as well as the dose to anyone else in the vicinity.

QUESTIONS FOR DISCUSSION AND CRITICAL THINKING

1. Compare natural background radiation with human-made radiation and describe the greatest source of each.
2. Explain the importance of understanding the measurement of radiation and dose limits.
3. Describe the two main photon–tissue interactions that occur in diagnostic radiography.
4. Compare short-term with long-term effects of exposure to ionizing radiation.
5. Relate time, distance, and shielding to patient radiation dose.
6. Discuss the best ways of keeping your radiation dose as low as possible.
7. Explain the use of a personal dosimeter.
8. Discuss the importance of keeping radiation dose to the population as low as reasonably achievable.

BIBLIOGRAPHY

Bushong S. *Radiologic science for technologists.* ed 11. St. Louis: Elsevier; 2017.
Callaway W. *Mosby's comprehensive review of radiography.* ed 7. St. Louis: Elsevier; 2017.

Lampignano J, Kendrick L. *Bontrager's textbook of radiographic positioning and related anatomy.* ed 9. St. Louis: Elsevier; 2018.
Long B, Rollins J, Smith B. *Merrill's atlas of radiographic positioning and procedures.* ed 14. St. Louis: Elsevier; 2020.
Sherer M, Visconti P, Ritenour R, Haynes K. *Radiation protection in medical radiography.* ed 8. St. Louis: Elsevier; 2018.

11

Ethics, Professionalism, and Law in Radiologic Technology

OBJECTIVES

On completion of this chapter, you should be able to:
- Interact with patients, peers, and professionals in a civil and considerate manner.
- Explain what is meant by professional confidentiality.
- Describe effective communication techniques.
- Discuss the procedures for protecting patient modesty and self-esteem.
- Explain how to project a professional image in attire and conduct.
- Discuss personal obligations that radiologic technologists have to their patients, to their profession, and to the society at large.
- Discuss the impact of medical malpractice on society.
- Define *tort* and explain its several forms in the health profession.
- Discuss patient consent rights and the radiologic technologist's role in ensuring the validity of the consent.
- Define *respondeat superior* and explain its significance in radiology services.
- Define *res ipsa loquitur* and explain how it may apply in radiology.
- List seven reasons why a radiologic technologist may be named as a defendant in a malpractice case.
- Discuss the steps a radiologic technologist may take to prevent a lawsuit against a health care provider.
- Discuss the importance of maintaining patient privacy.

OUTLINE

Initial Considerations
Professional Goals
Interpersonal Relationships
The Patient
    Patient Attitudes and Reactions
    Patient Modesty
Communication
Professional Confidentiality
Professional Image
Personal Obligations
Medical Malpractice

Torts
    Intentional Misconduct
    Unintentional Misconduct (Negligence)
Patient Consent
Respondeat Superior
Res Ipsa Loquitur
Legal Considerations of a Radiologic Technologist
Legal and Ethical Considerations Regarding new
   Technology
Conclusion

KEY TERMS

attitudes
case law
civil assault
civil battery
confidentiality
creeds

defendant
dignity
false imprisonment
modesty
moral
negligence

personal obligation
plaintiff
res ipsa loquitur
respondeat superior
standards of conduct
torts

INITIAL CONSIDERATIONS

By now you have realized that in addition to developing technical knowledge and skills, the foundation of radiologic technology encompasses **standards of conduct** and ideals essential to meeting both the emotional and physical needs of patients.

Radiologic technology encompasses a variety of specialties and plays an invaluable role in the practice of medicine. This service department provides vital information about the structure and function—both normal and abnormal—of the human body, and this information enables physicians to make accurate diagnoses to pursue care and treatment. Practitioners of this art and science play a key role in the total spectrum of health care services.

Those of you entering radiologic or other imaging technologies directly from high school may find that your age (youth) presents some problems. Typically, the general public questions the character and competence of anyone to whom they must entrust their care and treatment. With each new patient, your abilities and purposes may be on trial simply because of your age. A majority of patients may be senior citizens. To understand their opinions and standards, you must realize that, when they were young people, the people, experiences, and events of several decades ago influenced them. External influences temper attitudes from generation to generation. The degree of social freedom has changed considerably over the past few decades, and older generations may have difficulty believing that today's youth can measure up to the ethical and moral standards associated with the medical professions over the years. Your work and your conduct will prove them right or wrong.

Individuals who are entering this profession must ask themselves questions such as, "What do I expect from this field as a professional career?" and "What do I have to contribute?" to conduct a thorough self-analysis. Diagnostic imaging, whatever the chosen modality, is a service profession. Do you have a service-oriented personality? Will you be able to work with people who may be experiencing some of the worst situations in their lives, and can you do so with empathy? You need to consider the extremes that can occur. Unfortunately, through television and the many programs associated with medicine, dramatic license has taken over, and reality becomes overshadowed and somewhat glamorized. If you are expecting glamour and high drama, you may need to reconsider. The work will be demanding both physically and emotionally, and it entails a serious responsibility. If you are choosing correctly, the work will be immensely rewarding through the many people that you will help during their pain and illness.

PROFESSIONAL GOALS

In establishing a worthwhile goal, you must first view your chosen profession as more than a job. You should not pursue a simple goal of just passing a series of examinations and eventually becoming certified by the Registry or just earning a degree; instead, you should set a goal that will establish you as a first-rate professional. Imaging technology does not need dropouts or those unable to cope with the advances in the profession. What caliber of radiologic technologist would you prefer to care for you or your family? Certainly, you would want the services of a professional radiologic technologist—a combination of superior technical knowledge and skills applied in an understanding, caring, and compassionate manner—who works in harmony and cooperation with peers, physicians, radiologists, and all other hospital personnel.

Suppose that you, like many others, plan to use radiologic technology as a stepping stone in your long-range career plans to achieve some higher vocational goal. Does this mean that you need not apply yourself with as much dedication and effort as if radiologic technology were your ultimate professional goal? Definitely not. The needs are still the same. Whether you plan to pursue this profession for a temporary or indefinite length of time, respect it and respect yourself by excelling at all times.

INTERPERSONAL RELATIONSHIPS

If you enter the field of radiologic technology, you will encounter many individuals who will influence your education and training. First are the didactic and clinical instructors who are knowledgeable and skilled professionals; they are dedicated to assisting and guiding you to become a first-rate radiologic technologist, but the rest is up to you. The success of your learning experience depends primarily on your own incentive, dedication, and personal application.

As you contemplate entering this profession, you need to consider both your short- and long-term plans. Medical imaging has and will continue to develop very rapidly in its complexity. Are you interested in staying with and developing your knowledge and skills in keeping up with these changes to excel in this field? The goal of health care does not change except to become more efficient in its delivery and more successful in diagnosing and providing treatment. If this excellence in knowledge and skill is accompanied by an underlying desire to provide care and empathy for patients, the goal of service is being well served. Consider whether this is the reason that a career in medical imaging appeals to you.

If you are viewing this profession as a short-term goal, you may be shortchanging both yourself and the field.

You may limit yourself in the heights that you could achieve and what you would contribute to the field. If you are using this field as a stepping stone to a more advanced medical profession, you must apply yourself to learn everything you can in your academic and clinical experience to serve as a basis. However, those of us who have spent many decades as technologists and have grown with the field would hope that your plans and sense of dedication would become long range, that you would strive to excel beyond the basic requirements, and that you would become one of the building blocks of this profession.

You need to understand your instructors and their motivations. They may seem regimented in committing you to unmerciful schedules of study and practice, but they, too, have a goal to achieve. Within the 2 or 4 years that seem so long to you, they must teach you a large body of knowledge and assist you in developing your skills simply to meet the minimum standards. They must also try to motivate you to take part in additional studies, research, writing, and practice on your own. Their goal is to have you develop into a professional radiologic technologist; thus your association with your instructors should be one of mutual understanding and cooperative efforts in developing your professional education and training. You may find some comfort in knowing that your instructors—registered technologists, physicians, and radiologists—are all caught up in a process similar to yours; that is, they are constantly striving to keep abreast of continual advances in the field of medicine and related health services. All of these professional individuals represent your sources of information and learning. Take advantage of their assistance at every available opportunity.

Attending physicians and radiologists you encounter may appear to be distant, preoccupied, and generally indifferent to your presence in the department. You will find some to be exactly that; others will be a tremendous source of information and assistance with a friendly interest in your progress. Unfortunately, the wide gap between professional standings of the medical and technical fields continues; however, this gap can be bridged as each succeeding generation of radiologic technologists exhibits increasingly higher levels of knowledge, skill, and personal professionalism. Radiologic technologists need to assert themselves as essential members of the total health service team.

Success in the health care industry and in the treatment of patients depends not only on the physicians but also on the total team effort of health care professionals; this includes radiologic technologists, other imaging specialists, and nurses to provide the total information needed for a diagnosis and proper course of treatment for the patient. In the past, physicians were at the top of the pyramid. Although the physician still makes the final decision about the course of treatment, this determination is based on findings of the associated professions working as a team. Always keep in mind that your work as an imaging professional makes an important contribution to the team effort; you can take pride in carrying out such a serious responsibility. Without imaging technology services, diagnoses and effective patient care and treatment would be extremely difficult and, in many instances, impossible.

THE PATIENT

When continuing to consider the individuals involved in the course of education and training, we must discuss the patients. How important are they and why? Suppose somebody built a hospital, furnished it with the most advanced equipment, and staffed it with a full complement of all professionals—and then no patients came. Now the picture comes into focus! The patient is the object of all the attentions and efforts to detect injuries, diagnose diseases, and deliver treatments.

Who becomes a patient? Each and every member of the human race is a potential patient. Patients come in various shapes, sizes, ages, colors, **creeds**, religions, and politics. Illness, injury, and disease play no favorites and make no exceptions. The patient is someone's child, sibling, parent, friend, or mate. Each patient is important to someone, and all patients are important; their physical comfort, emotional security, and confidence in an individual who can help them all need to be considered equally.

Your focus must always be on what you can contribute to help this individual who needs your particular service. Your personal attitude toward your patient, your work, and your work environment must be a desire to make your contribution the very best within your responsibilities. In working with students over many decades, one fundamental issue has been the attitude of the student, and this attitude would or would not propel a student to excel in his or her work. The patient senses this attitude, and so do colleagues, instructors, and others. A person with a positive, energetic, and caring attitude will always be a winner; all other issues can be overcome through study, experience, and continuing education.

Patient Attitudes and Reactions

What circumstances influence the **attitudes** (i.e., feelings, emotions) and actions of a patient who is entering a hospital? Except when it is for childbirth, entering the hospital is not usually a happy occasion. Hospitalization usually involves pain and fear caused by an injury, illness, or disease; the prognosis can be questionable or hopeless. Emotional reactions may appear magnified or even irrational, and the radiographic technologist needs to interact with them in an appropriate manner. Fears can be alleviated by a caring, positive approach and an understanding of your patients' concerns. Health care workers who are positive and encouraging, who can work with the negative or defeatist patient, and who are able to elevate a patient's level of stability and comfort are exceptional.

A patient may react by reaffirming or intensifying religious beliefs and practices. Religion is a private, personal matter. You must respect each patient's choice of worship. Religion may be a patient's bid for security or a last hope and source of strength to endure whatever lies ahead. You are not to judge the merits of anyone's religion or to promote the merits of your own; simply respect the right of choice. Sometimes life throws a curve, making the ability to remain neutral a challenge. You are reminded that radiologic imaging is a service profession and that you cannot choose your patients. As a true professional, you must be able to interact with any and all individuals without prejudice.

Just as you should not become involved in religious differences, you should also be impartial when encountering patients of a different race, color, nationality, or gender identification. Each patient is entitled to the highest degree of care and concern that you are able to provide. As a health service practitioner dedicated to saving lives, how could you do otherwise?

Unfortunately, societies' problems, prejudices, and attitudes can be brought into the hospital or clinic by our patients; these can be diminished or amplified by our response to the patients and their particular needs. Outside of the hospital walls, people are generally focused on daily activities and pleasures within their own personal spheres. However, when pain, illness, and trauma enter our lives, we all become equal. Thus, as a medical professional, you will need to recognize and be able to deal with many socioeconomic, ethnic, and religious differences and to treat all patients with equal respect. In summary, you should serve each patient with equal care and dedication.

Patient Modesty

As we continue to consider the patient, we come to the important responsibility of respecting and preserving the patient's **modesty**. All people value their bodies as part of their total person and deserve to have them managed in a respectful manner. The degree of modesty exhibited by a patient may vary from extreme modesty to a total lack of it. You must observe the rules of draping and covering the patient to the greatest extent possible, depending on the examination. As a professional, you may find yourself in a delicate situation that requires you to decide whether you are the most suitable technologist to perform an examination on a certain patient. If an examination requires a

position that could be embarrassing to patients, you should use considerable tact with these patients to preserve modesty and personal **dignity**.

Traditionally, older generations seem to find some of the actions, dress (or lack of dress), and attitudes of the younger generations alarming and possibly distasteful; you can probably expect to encounter many such people during your training. Patients who would find it comfortable at the beach or at a social event may shun having their bodies exposed or touched by a stranger, even one who is a medical professional. Compared with these other, more regular activities, the issue here is one of loss of choice or control. Therefore, treat every patient as if each were modest. This consideration is the patient's right and your responsibility. If you do this, patients will be most appreciative, and they will recognize that you are truly a professional to be trusted.

COMMUNICATION

Effective communication is a technique that you need to master, and you need to recognize that it includes verbal communication, facial expressions, and other body language. Your attitude, the tone of your voice, your appearance and dress, and your facial expressions combine to present a first impression to the patient. This impression can be positive or negative and can either increase their anxieties or instill confidence that they can expect high-quality, efficient, and caring service from you. As a health care service provider, you must always endeavor to first build the patient's trust in your abilities. Patients must be able to sense your professionalism, and they will respond positively and with confidence to your care.

How you divulge information and what information you share—whether fact or opinion, intentionally or inadvertently—could cause a patient considerable anguish. Your first responsibility is to converse with the patient in an intelligent, professional manner that is pleasant and courteous. A patient who is under stress may be decidedly unpleasant to you at times. However, you must maintain control over your emotions, remain pleasant, and try to alleviate the patient's apprehensions, which may be causing or contributing to the unpleasant behavior. During your initial contact with a particular patient, you must be able to determine what would be the most appropriate manner in which to interact with him or her. The patient should leave your care feeling that you were interested and had performed your best service at all times.

PROFESSIONAL CONFIDENTIALITY

One of the major restrictions that the health care profession imposes on you is the need to maintain strict **confidentiality** of medical and personal information about a patient. The patient may ask about his or her condition; however, this information cannot be revealed by the technologist to the patient, the patient's family, or others outside the department without the direct consent of the patient's physician. Breach of confidence is one of the major problems encountered when providing patient care and can result in legal problems for the department and hospital. Information should not be discussed throughout the hospital with other department personnel except in the direct line of duty when requested from one ancillary department to another or with nursing service to meet specific medical needs. Information should never be discussed with your own family or friends in even the most general terms; doing so violates the patient's rights and damages both the department and the hospital's reputations. Your instructors will emphasize and reiterate the need to maintain strict confidence of information about patients, the department, and the hospital. Consider how you would feel if you were the patient and your private information were the topic of a conversation down the hall, during a coffee break in the cafeteria, or anywhere in public. Patient and medical record confidentiality is legally governed by the Health Insurance Portability and Accountability Act (HIPAA) of 1996.

You are responsible for knowing all of the rules and regulations concerning the patient rights involved in the provision of health care services. Preservation of patient confidentiality is still a vital issue and is challenged in court virtually every day in some part of the country. The patient's condition or any personal information, including a particular diagnostic examination, must be held in strictest confidence; this right also applies to any public figures and officials. Discuss any changes that involve providing medical services with your instructors to ensure that you do not inadvertently violate a public trust.

PROFESSIONAL IMAGE

In developing your professional image, you need to consider another area that is often contested: specific standards for dress and grooming. You should keep in mind that the patient's first impression of you is strongly influenced by your personal appearance, including your facial expressions. Before the first word is spoken, patients begin to formulate an opinion of you, the person to whom they must entrust themselves during the course of radiography or other procedures that you may perform. The dress and grooming of the staff and the appearance of the department and the hospital influence an immediate opinion. For example, we are exposed to visible body piercing jewelry (e.g., in the nose, tongue, lips, and eyebrows). Although such extremes may be acceptable during high school and

college, they are not readily acceptable in professional medical circles. A high percentage of your patients will be of older generations or of certain ethnic or religious persuasions that may find extremes in dress and jewelry unacceptable or even offensive. Regardless of the sterling character of the radiologic technologist, professional image is essential.

We work with the individual rights of both the patient and the health care professional. In this instance, the patient will have a preconceived idea of how the health care worker should look and act, and as the patient-customer, his or her right is paramount. The total picture of the radiologic technologist should be one of neatness, cleanliness, and friendly efficiency if the patient is to gain any confidence in the type of treatment that can be expected. Always keep in mind the patient's image of what a professional should look like.

As social attitudes have changed and the manner of dress and grooming have become more casual, these attitudes have carried over into the hospital environment with uniform and grooming codes becoming more lenient. However, no argument is going to change the fact that a casual appearance does not epitomize a technically skilled, highly motivated, and competent radiologic technologist— a professional health care specialist. A professional image of hospital personnel has been perpetuated in the public mind over the years, and changes in ideals of this nature are not readily accepted. The hospital establishes dress and grooming codes appropriate to the hospital environment, and you are expected to adhere to these codes regardless of personal tastes.

In the past few years when casual Friday was introduced in the business community, the same was soon introduced into the hospital environment. Although widely accepted in other fields, casual wear in the hospital gives the impression of a casual attitude and a lessening in professionalism in the eyes of older-generation patients and patients of various ethnic and religious groups. Patients' concerns are not casual, and they could be discouraged about the quality of service and care they may receive if the hospital personnel are not dressed to the professional level that patients have come to expect. Although this may seem unfair, it is the reality, and the patients' needs come first. The rationale is sound and in the best interest of good rapport between the patient and working professionals. You must be willing to accept it.

PERSONAL OBLIGATIONS

What are your personal, professional, and ethical obligations to the art and science of radiologic technology? You are legally responsible for your actions, even as a student. The second half of this chapter discusses legal aspects in greater detail. You are protected in part by being limited to basic responsibilities under supervision in early training. As your skills and knowledge increase, this degree of supervision will diminish, and personal responsibility will increase. As a graduate, you will become totally responsible, from the moral and legal standpoint, to adhere to the rules and standards that you have been taught.

By now, you should realize that radiologic technology must be more than just a job to you. Can you accept the personal obligation to pursue continuing education and to grow in the knowledge and skills of a constantly advancing field so that you will not rapidly become obsolete and second rate? Do you feel motivated to participate in and support the activities of the professional organizations that have student members so that you can master the new advancements in the field?

To become proficient and a leader in your field, you must demand the highest quality in your classes and clinical experience. In this way, you will develop professionally and advance the stature of the profession among the health service fields. Success can be measured by what you have accomplished technically, by the manner in which you interact with your patients and the rest of the health care staff, and by your personal contributions to writings and research.

Each profession has leaders and followers; radiologic technology is no exception. However, many dedicated leaders have developed and nurtured a professional organization that is worthy of your respect and support. The typical leader expends more than the minimal effort required to survive by motivating others to achieve competent, professional performance.

The professional survival rate among radiologic technologists has decreased as they try to outlast the new information, techniques, and equipment that rapidly render them obsolete in the field. To succeed, you must believe in the merits of the profession and its growing importance in health care. For many, radiologic technology has been a short-term career with a high attrition rate because they lacked the incentive, determination, and personal effort to succeed. Radiologic technology is, in fact, one of the most exciting and challenging health care fields today; it is a scientific wonder that allows the structure and function of every cell and organ of the body to be studied by the human eye and mind. Today, a radiologic technologist who keeps abreast of the field must be an exceptional individual—a technologist, a scientist, and a humanitarian.

Lapses in ethics, patient confidentiality, standards of care, or professional judgment often lead to legal issues in the clinical environment. This branch of law is often referred to a medicolegal. The American society in which we live and work as health care professionals is "a nation ruled by laws, not by men." This quote suggests that law establishes the relationship not only between the individual and the government but also between individuals. The dominant power over our lives is not the authority of a king, junta, or popularly elected president. Rather, political power is embodied in a complex system that is known simply as "the law."

Law is not a single entity; it is a composite body of customs, practices, and rules. In our society, these rules and practices come from the federal and state constitutions, the statutes of both state and federal legislatures, regulations issued by the administrative agencies of the executive branch of government, and the interpretations of these constitutions, statutes, and regulations that are rendered by the courts. The law that arises from the courts' interpretations of these constitutions, statutes, and regulations is known as case law. Community values generally inform and shape the rules formed by particular administrations, legislatures, and courts. However, any reading of contemporary affairs makes the notion clear that perceived community values and our laws are not always in agreement. The history of law—in all forms—is a history of accumulating wisdom and experience that is mixed with substantial amounts of give and take among all segments of society.

The underlying motivation for all forms of law is to protect people and property, to provide for correcting injustice, and to compensate for injury. The specific area of the law that most concerns health practitioners is known as medical malpractice.

MEDICAL MALPRACTICE

You probably know about large medical malpractice awards to injured patients. Even large medical institutions can be financially devastated when they are required to pay such amounts. To reduce the risk of such medical malpractice awards, you should understand the nature of the legal relationship between the individual patient and health care providers.

The legal rights that exist between the individual patient and those who provide health care to that patient are essentially the same rights that exist between any two individuals, with some significant exceptions. One of these exceptions is that, unlike two individuals who act on roughly equal footing to transact the sale of property or to enter business contracts, the relationship between a patient and a health care provider is rarely that of two equals. Because society has allowed physicians to practice medicine, it also imposes on them the duty to conduct that practice according to accepted standards. In effect, along with special privilege must go special responsibility. Failure to meet this special responsibility can leave a physician or other health care practitioner such as a radiologic technologist open to lawsuits alleging wrongful or negligent acts that result in injury to a patient. The law refers to such wrongful or negligent acts generally as *torts*.

TORTS

Torts are not easy to define, but a basic distinction is that they are violations of civil, as opposed to criminal, law. However, the same conduct may constitute both a tort and a violation of the criminal law. Intentionally punching someone in the nose without consent or excuse would constitute both a civil battery (a tort) and a crime. If the victim brought a civil tort action against the perpetrator, the perpetrator could be required to pay money damages directly to the victim to compensate for any injury to the victim. If the state brought a criminal action, the perpetrator could suffer a prison sentence or other punishment for that conduct.

For this discussion, we can also say that tort law is personal injury law. Torts include specific conditions in which the law allows for compensation to be paid to an individual when that individual is damaged or injured by another.

Two types of torts have been defined: (1) those resulting from intentional action and (2) those resulting from unintentional action.

Intentional Misconduct

Several situations can occur in which a tort action can be brought against the health professional because of some action that was deliberately taken.

1. A tort of **civil assault** can be filed if a patient is reasonably fearful of being injured by the imprudent conduct of the radiologic technologist. If found liable, the radiologic technologist could be held responsible for providing financial compensation to the patient for damages.
2. A tort of **civil battery** would be an appropriate proceeding when actual bodily harm has been inflicted on a patient as a result of intentional physical contact between a health care provider and a patient, again with potential for liability against the radiologic technologist. A health worker cannot touch a patient for any reason unless a valid consent is given by the patient to receive medical care. (The elements that are required for a valid consent are discussed later.)
3. Other forms of intentional misconduct include invasion of privacy; defamation, whether spoken (slander) or written (libel); and false imprisonment. An example of invasion of privacy is when a radiologic technologist publicly discusses privileged and confidential information obtained from the attending physician or the patient's medical record. An example of **false** **imprisonment** would be unnecessarily confining or restraining the patient without the patient's permission. If during the performance of a radiographic examination, a patient is strapped to the table or similarly confined without having given permission to be so restricted, that patient would have grounds for a charge of false imprisonment.

Unintentional Misconduct (Negligence)

If the determination is made that a health care provider acted negligently, he or she may be held liable for specific actions that cause injury to patients, even though the actions were unintentional. Negligence can be the basis for tort action because the radiologic technologist, although intending to help, actually caused damage by failing to perform as the patient and the employing hospital had the right to expect that person to perform.

As is the case in the majority of American legal principles, the idea of negligence as a basis for civil liability came from English common law. The concepts of medical negligence and liability have a long history, dating at least to the fourteenth century. We have written records that in 1373, Justice John Cavendish decided the case of *Stratton v Swanlond* with the conclusion that if the patient was harmed as a consequence of the physician's negligence, that physician should be held liable. Justice Cavendish added that if the physician did all that could be done, the physician should not be held liable, even if no cure was obtained. More than 500 years ago, the basic ingredients of negligence and liability were expressed in an English-language court.

Negligence can be defined as a breach or a failure to fulfill an expected standard of care. Generally, the standard of care required is that degree of care that would be used by a "reasonable person" under the circumstances. For health care professionals, however, the standard of care is modified somewhat and is determined by the degree of care or skill that a reasonable health care professional would exercise under the circumstances. This definition means that the radiologic technologist owes a duty to the patient based on the standard of care that a reasonable radiologic technologist is expected to provide under similar circumstances.

The "reasonable person" and the "reasonable radiologic technologist" discussed earlier do not refer to any particular person but rather to a hypothetical reasonable person and reasonable radiologic technologist. Thus, a person described by everyone as "reasonable" will still be liable for negligence if, in a particular situation, he or she fails to act as the hypothetical reasonable person would have acted. For example, if a person exceeds the speed limit and causes an accident, that person will still be guilty of negligence, even if six very reasonable people are found to testify that they sometimes exceed the speed limit. The hypothetical reasonable person never exceeds the speed limit. Thus, normal and reasonable people are often found negligent in particular circumstances. Failure to perform to this expected standard of care will constitute negligence and result in liability.

For a health care professional to be found negligent in a court and subsequently held liable for damages, the civil proceeding must establish the following elements:

1. That a *duty* of care (or standard of care) was owed by the radiologic technologist to the patient
2. That a *breach* of that duty occurred by the radiologic technologist
3. That the *cause* of injury was the radiologic technologist's negligence
4. That the *injury* to the patient actually occurred

Each of these elements is discussed below:

1. *The standard of care owed to the injured person.* The radiologic technologist must exercise the care that a reasonable radiologic technologist is expected to exercise under the same circumstances. If a physician instructs radiographer Boswell to radiograph patient Abbott's right leg, Boswell has a duty to radiograph Abbott's right leg properly. If Boswell radiographs Abbott's right leg, Boswell will have performed as a reasonable and prudent radiographer would have acted under similar circumstances. If, however, Boswell radiographs Abbott's *left* leg, Boswell is breaching the standard of care by failing to follow the physician's directions. Boswell does not have a duty to exercise care above and beyond what a reasonable radiographer would exercise. For example, Boswell does not have the responsibility to repair broken bones that are discovered while radiographing patient Abbott. Evidence about what the standard of care should be usually consists of the testimony of an expert witness, such as a competent radiographer or radiologist. Testimony will concentrate on what conduct would be reasonably expected under the circumstance based on customarily accepted standards within the medical community.

2. *Breach of the standard of care.* A breach is failure to exercise reasonable care. What if Boswell radiographs the right leg but the quality of that radiograph is not adequate to provide diagnostic information? If a radiographer has the duty to ensure that radiographs are clear and of the highest quality for the physician's diagnosis, then giving the physician an inadequate radiograph is a breach of the radiographer's duty. If a patient's condition deteriorates because the physician could not properly interpret the radiograph, then the patient would have grounds to sue the physician and the radiographer. How inadequate need a radiograph be before a jury would declare the technologist in breach of duty? This question is difficult and is one that would be resolved in court with the assistance of expert witnesses and by the judgment of a jury on a case-by-case basis.

3. *The radiographer's negligence must be shown to be the direct cause of the patient's injury.* The breach of duty must be the factual cause of the injury. If the radiographer has the duty to make sure that a dizzy or semiconscious patient does not fall from the examination table, it would be a breach of that duty if the radiographer left the room. If, on the radiographers leaving the room, the patient fell from the table and sustained injuries, a jury hearing the tort action would likely agree that the radiographer's breach of duty (negligence) *caused* the injuries; this judgment is reached because leaving the room would be closely related to the patient's falling from the table. Suppose, however, that the radiographer leaves the room and on return finds that the patient is very upset that the radiographer left the room, although the patient did not fall off the table. Days later, the patient is standing in the hall telling his wife that the radiologic technologist had left him alone while he was semiconscious on the examination table. In describing the incident, the patient becomes upset, faints, and, as a result, fractures an arm. The patient might argue that the radiographer caused the fractured arm. The patient probably would not prevail in court, however, because he or she would have difficulty proving that the radiologic technologist's action was a "proximate cause" of the fractured arm. If the cause of injury is too remote from the breach of duty (the negligence), even though factual cause seems evident, then the negligence is not the proximate cause of injury.

4. *The patient sustains actual injury.* A personal injury case or tort will not be successful in establishing liability if no damages occur. If a patient falls from an examination table because the radiographer leaves the room but does not incur any injuries, the patient cannot expect to receive compensation.

Applying the negligence standard to Boswell's error in radiographing the patient's left leg instead of the right is relatively easy. Obviously, a reasonable radiologic technologist would x-ray the correct limb.

Examples

In real life, applying the negligence standard is not always as easy, as the following examples demonstrate. These examples are based loosely on real cases. Some facts have been changed to maintain the privacy of persons involved.

Case 1. An older adult patient was admitted to the hospital for treatment and tests. She was sent to the radiology department for a routine chest x-ray examination. While standing at the chest unit, she fell and broke her hip. The patient filed suit against the hospital, the referring physician, the radiologists, and the technologist. In the lawsuit, the patient claimed that these parties acted negligently, that she should have been supported or restrained while being radiographed, and that the physician should have noted her tendency to become dizzy on the examination request.

In this case, the patient was able to prove that she had a tendency to become dizzy and that the physician knew about it. The evidence in the case also showed that the physician's examination request had no reference to the patient's tendency to become dizzy.

The radiologist and technologist brought forth evidence that the examination and x-ray process were conducted in a manner that was customary, reasonable, and generally accepted in the medical community. They were also able to show that they had no knowledge of the patient's tendency to become dizzy. Accordingly, the radiologist and technologist were able to convince the jury that they were not negligent.

On the other hand, the jury found that the referring physician was negligent for not noting the patient's tendency to become dizzy on the request form. The jury believed that this breached the physician's standard of care and that this breach caused the patient's injury.

Questions and Comments. By adding facts or slightly changing the facts, the result of this case might be different. For instance, if the physician had noted the patient's tendency to become dizzy on the examination request, the jury probably would have held the radiologist and technologist liable and excused the referring physician. The case also might have been decided differently if the hospital had a policy of restraining all patients during the x-ray process (with the patient's consent) and if the radiologist and technologist had violated that policy.

How do you think the case would have turned out if no notations were made on the examination request but the radiologist or technologist had noticed the patient walking unsteadily before the x-ray? Would it matter if this observation occurred 2 days before the x-ray? Five minutes before the x-ray? Why?

Case 2. A hospitalized patient was scheduled for an emergency radiographic examination that required the injection of a contrast medium. The floor nurse inserted the needle into the vein, and the patient was transported to the radiology department. In the radiology department, the contrast medium was injected; however, the needle was not in the vein when the contrast media was injected. This situation resulted in extravasation and serious damage to the tissue surrounding the vessel. The patient sued, among others, the hospital, the nurse, and the technologist. The suit was settled before trial, and the hospital made a substantial settlement payment to the patient.

Questions and Comments. This case illustrates a real-life example of *res ipsa loquitur* (defined later in this chapter). The circumstances suggest that the injury simply would not have occurred in the absence of negligence by someone. Thus, to avoid liability, each of the defendants must prove that he or she was not the cause of the negligence. Accordingly, if the case were tried, the nurse would attempt to prove that he or she properly inserted the needle in the vein and that the needle became dislodged after the patient left the floor. On the other hand, the technologist would attempt to show that the needle was not inserted correctly in the first place.

The case also raises the question of whether the technologist, having learned venipuncture in school, should have been the one to determine the proper placement of the needle. As previously discussed, however, the standard of care is subject to evolution and change. The patient might have convinced a jury that a reasonably experienced technologist should have a duty to determine the proper placement of the needle. If the jury agreed, the standard of care for technologists might well be increased to include the duty to make such determinations.

These comments are not intended to suggest what the standard of care for technologists is or ought to be in this situation; rather, they are designed to demonstrate the complexity of the "negligence" concept and to stimulate thinking about how law (i.e., the standard of care) could evolve and influence society (e.g., schools and educators) and vice versa.

Case 3. This case takes a different twist because the technologist is not the defendant but the plaintiff. In this case, the technologist sued his employer, alleging that he had developed chronic granulocytic leukemia as a result of overexposure to radiation. The technologist testified that he had to support patients daily while the patients were being radiographed and that this subjected him to radiation exposure. The technologist stated that he could not use proper restraining devices because of the large number of patients he was required to move through the radiology department. He also testified that lead aprons, shields, and gloves were not always easily available to him.

In this case, the judge found the hospital negligent and awarded damages to the technologist relating to his leukemia. The judge believed that the hospital did not take reasonable precautions to limit the exposure of technologists to radiation.

Questions and Comments. This case presents several interesting issues. It might well have been decided differently by a different judge or jury. For instance, some courts or juries might have determined that the technologist's own negligence (i.e., not insisting on using lead shields, aprons, and gloves) contributed to the disease.

The case also had the potential of presenting causation problems for the technologist. What if the technologist also had a heart condition and such a condition contributed to his injuries? What if the hospital had produced evidence that the leukemia could have been caused by factors other than exposure to radiation?

In any event, this case illustrates the need for technologists to take appropriate precautions to prevent unnecessary exposure to radiation and for hospitals to make appropriate equipment available and to enforce procedures designed to reduce unnecessary exposure.

PATIENT CONSENT

The general rule is that patients have the right to consent to or refuse anything that is done to them in the hospital. Patient consent can be written, oral, or implied. Implied consent would be used in circumstances in which a patient is unconscious in an emergency department; the assumption is that the patient would want to give consent to receive needed care. The patient can revoke consent at any time. Even if the patient has previously granted verbal consent, written consent, or implied consent, at no time can a patient be denied the right to withdraw consent. For consent to be valid, three conditions must be met:

1. The patient must be of legal age and mentally competent.
2. The patient must offer consent voluntarily.
3. The patient must be adequately informed about the medical care being recommended. Because adequate information about treatment is generally known only by the physician or the health care provider, special responsibility is required to ensure that the patient understands the type of care and the potential risks that are being considered. Thus, you should accurately explain to your patients any procedure you will perform and what you expect of that patient.

RESPONDEAT SUPERIOR

The doctrine of *respondeat superior*, which is a Latin phrase that means "let the master answer," requires that an employer pay the victim for the torts committed by its employees. If a radiologic technologist is employed by a hospital, the hospital can be held jointly liable for whatever the radiologic technologist might do in a negligent manner. An injured patient does not have to prove that the hospital was negligent, only that the radiologic technologist was liable. Because the hospital employs the radiologic technologist, the hospital is automatically held jointly liable. Although the employing hospital may be jointly liable with an employee, this ruling does not mean that a radiologic technologist is immune from damage suits or relieved of personal responsibility for breach of duty. All people are responsible for their own injurious conduct.

RES IPSA LOQUITUR

In most tort cases, the **plaintiff** (the injured person bringing the suit) has the responsibility of proving that the **defendant** (the person being sued) should be held liable. Certain cases of negligence exist, however, in which the defendant is required to prove innocence. *Res ipsa loquitur* is a Latin phrase that means "the thing speaks for itself." The doctrine of *res ipsa loquitur* applies to a case that is built around evidence demonstrating that an injury could not have occurred if no negligence existed. An example of such a case would be one in which the discovery is made that a pair of forceps has been left in the patient's abdomen after surgery. They were not in the patient before surgery, and they could be in the patient only as a result of negligence on the part of the surgical team. As another example, a patient's being exposed to radiation sufficient to cause skin lesions could result only from negligence on the part of the radiologic technologist. In these cases, the procedures begin with the facts of evidence and proceed to establish that these facts would not have been true if negligence had not existed on someone's part. In these circumstances, the defendants must demonstrate that they were not the party responsible for the negligent act.

Patients may be harmed in ways other than physical, and one way is failure to maintain patient confidentiality. Divulging a patient's condition or other information contained in a patient's medical record could cause financial loss or social embarrassment to the patient. Accordingly, strict laws and policies exist to protect patients' privacy and the confidentiality of their medical records. Maintaining patient privacy is a significant issue not only because failure to do so may harm the patient, but also because such failure will expose the caregiver and employer to embarrassing, time-consuming lawsuits and the risk of financial loss and other sanctions.

Generally speaking, patients' medical records (their radiographs are a part of the medical records) belong to the hospital or institution where their care was given. However, the information contained in the records belongs to the patient. Without the patient's consent, this information cannot be divulged or released to anyone else. Certain exceptions to this rule exist, such as releasing information in response to a valid court order, but the exceptions are very limited. You should consult the applicable laws of your jurisdiction and the specific policies of your employer before making any patient disclosure. A caregiver can be liable for disclosing patient information even if the disclosure is unintentional or inadvertent and even if the caregiver honestly believed the disclosure would not harm the patient. This consideration is important while working with patients during your clinical practice.

LEGAL CONSIDERATIONS OF A RADIOLOGIC TECHNOLOGIST

Although the radiologic technologist does not encounter anywhere near the number of malpractice suits that are directed against physicians, a radiologic technologist might be held liable for several reasons. Saundra Warner, a distinguished radiologic educator and attorney, lists seven reasons why a plaintiff's attorney might choose to name a radiologic technologist as a defendant:

1. To meet the conditions of *res ipsa loquitur*
2. Because the hospital or its physicians are immune from action or because the radiologic technologist is not directly controlled by the physician
3. Because the hospital or physicians or both cannot be sued as defendants because they are not directly negligent, and proximate causation cannot be applied to the hospital or physicians
4. Because of various trial tactics
5. To secure the radiologic technologist in pretrial testimony and as a witness in subsequent court testimony
6. Because the plaintiff presumes that the radiologic technologist has assets or insurance
7. Because it aids or is essential to the case

Maintaining records and documents of any procedure that you think is questionable or about which you might be asked to provide information is always prudent.

LEGAL AND ETHICAL CONSIDERATIONS REGARDING NEW TECHNOLOGY

Technology tends to develop faster than legal or ethical guidelines regarding its use. Automobiles, for example, were in use long before states passed laws requiring drivers to be licensed. New imaging technology must be proven to be safe. It must have the approval of the appropriate governing agencies before being cleared for use in clinical practice. Although most of this is beyond the scope of practice of a radiologic technologist, you should be aware that legal issues can arise from using technology that has not yet been proven to be safe and beneficial to the patient. Using only proven technology is also referred to in the *Standards of Ethics* of the American Registry of Radiologic Technologists.

As discussed in other chapters, continuing education is a requirement in your profession, and the issues raised in this chapter illustrate why. Technologists need to be aware of new technologies and related legal and ethical issues.

CONCLUSION

The objective of radiographic imaging is to produce images that are diagnostically sound and radiation safe. This objective requires that image quality be maintained at the highest level possible.

With the appropriate educational background and the determination to achieve, you can advance to the top of the radiologic technology field. When you practice professionalism and technical excellence, the patient will benefit, the health care community will benefit, and you will personally benefit. You will be one of many individuals working together to achieve the best possible treatment of injuries and diseases. Radiologic technology holds the key that has opened many doors for medical advancement, and the potential is still unlimited.

People now entering this profession are at the threshold of some of the most rapid advancements. Technologists who have been in the profession for several decades are in awe and look forward with great anticipation to future advancements in radiologic technology. Those of you entering this program are at the cutting edge of technology; you have the prospect for a strong future in this field and the chance to excel beyond your imagination.

At the same time, you have a duty to give high-quality care to your patients, and this duty includes not causing them injury. If you professionally apply your knowledge and training in radiologic technology, provide exemplary patient care, thoroughly explain procedures to your patients, work with extreme care, and question any abnormal instructions, you will probably never be involved in a lawsuit. However, being well-versed in medicolegal issues as presented in this chapter will assist you in avoiding situations that may compromise patient care and your clinical reputation.

QUESTIONS FOR DISCUSSION AND CRITICAL THINKING

1. Discuss your goals as a new radiography student.
2. Describe the importance of establishing healthy relationships with everyone involved in your radiography education.
3. Given the aging of the patient population, explain the importance of clear communication and respect for modesty and privacy when caring for them.
4. Compare intentional misconduct with unintentional misconduct (negligence).
5. Discuss the four elements needed to prove negligence has occurred.
6. Describe the elements required for informed consent.
7. Explain *respondeat superior* and *res ips loquitur*.
8. Discuss the ways in which good practice can help prevent being involved in a malpractice lawsuit.

BIBLIOGRAPHY

American Hospital Association. Patient's Bill of Rights. Available at http://www.RadiologyToday.net.

Blaut JM. The medical malpractice crisis: its causes and future. *Ins Couns J.* 1977; 44:114.

Bundy A. *Radiology and the law.* Rockville, MD: Aspen; 1988.

Church EJ. Legal trends in imaging. *Radiol Technol.* 2004; 76(1):31–45.

Comment. medico-legal implications of recent legislation concerning allied health practitioners, *Loy LAL Rev.* 1978; 11:379.

Greenberg v Michael Rees Hospital, 83 Ill 2d 282, 415 NE 2d 390 1981.

Hillcrest Medical Center v Wier, 373 P 2d 45 Okla, 1962.

Hospital Authority v Adams, 110 Ga App 848, 140 SE 2d 139 1964.

Johnson v Grant Hospital, 31 Ohio App 2d 118, 286 NE 2d 368 1968.

Keene v Methodist Hospital, 324 F Supp 233 1971.

Krayse v Bridgeport Hospital, 169 Conn 1, 362 A 2d 802 1975.

Mulholland HR. *The legal status of the hospital medical staff, St. Louis ULJ.* 1978; 22:485.

Prosser W. *Handbook of the law of torts.* ed 4. San Diego: Harcourt Brace Jovanovich; 1971.

Rose v Hakim, 345 F Supp 1300 1972.

Runyan v Goodrum, 228 SW 397 Ark 1921.

Simmons v South Shore Hospital, 340 Ill App 153, 91 NE 2d 135 1950.

Simpson v Sisters of Charity, 284 Or 547, 588 P 2d 4 1978.

Standefer v United States, 511 F 2d 101 1975.

Toth v Community Hospital, 22 NY 2d 255, 239 NE 368 1968.

Tucson General Hospital v Russell, 7 Ariz App 193, 437 P 2d 677 1968.

Warner SL. former assistant professor of radiology: Personal communication. In: *University of Maryland School of Medicine*; 1981.

12

Radiology Department:
Organization and Operation

OBJECTIVES

On completion of this chapter, you should be able to:
- Describe the role of a hospital administrator.
- Describe the role of a radiology administrator.
- Describe the role and function of a policy and procedures manual.
- List essential procedures and policy items included in a procedures manual.
- Describe the rationale for a quality assurance program.
- List the factors that determine the selection of radiology equipment.
- Contrast quality assurance with quality control.
- Explain equipment evaluation and monitoring.
- Explain the significance of a quality assurance program from the standpoint of patient care, economics, and staff development.

OUTLINE

Organization
    Radiology Staff Activities
Policies and Procedures
    Requesting Radiology Services
    Procedures Manual
    Human Resource Procedures
    Safety
    Sanitation and Infection Control
Reimbursement
    Prospective Payment for Medicare
Economics of Radiology
    Staffing

    Equipment
Quality Assurance and Quality Control
    Radiographic Equipment
    Radiographer
    Patients
    Creating Good Physical Conditions
    Maintaining Competency
    Administrative Evaluation
    Radiologist
    Maintaining Personal Standards
Conclusion

KEY TERMS

Affordable Care Act
compliance evaluations
exposure factors
flowcharts
hospital safety committee
life-cycle cost
Medicaid

Medicare
mobile (portable) unit
Occupational Safety and Health
    Administration (OSHA)
organizational charts
personnel monitoring
positioning skills

procedures manual
prospective payment system
quality assurance
radiation safety committee
scope of practice

You will soon be, or already are, spending a lot of time gaining clinical experience in a radiology department. Although you may also spend time in outpatient clinics, prompt care centers, or large practices for clinical experience, the bulk of your time will be in a traditional radiology department in a hospital.

The key to every successful radiology department is its dedication to serving people, with the patient being the most important person served along with the attending physicians. Without attending physicians and patients, there is no need for the radiology department. Such dedication to service must also include the working relationships among the radiologic technologists, the supervisors of the department, the radiologists, other hospital departments, and the hospital administration.

The characteristics of a radiology department are determined by the roles and functions of the hospital and the needs of the community it serves. If these facilities are part of a large teaching institution, some departments may have teaching and research in addition to patient care responsibilities.

Although no typical or average radiology department exists, certain characteristics are common to most departments. The organization of a radiology department affects its internal structure and the disposition and management of human and fiscal resources. Management goals are to arrange employees into working groups according to their work functions. Administration directs the efforts and skills of employees toward reaching departmental objectives in a cohesive and satisfying fashion.

Specialized areas within a radiology department may include diagnostic radiology, nuclear medicine, sonography, mammography, and interventional radiology. Large departments may also include radiation therapy.

This chapter is focused on the diagnostic radiology department because it is the largest and is the first clinical affiliation for the student. A radiology department may also be referred to as imaging department, department of imaging, department of medical imaging, or diagnostic radiology department.

ORGANIZATION

The hospital chief executive officer (CEO) and the medical staff are responsible for the operation of the hospital. The CEO is responsible for planning, developing, and maintaining programs that implement the policies and achieve the goals established by the governing body, normally a board of directors. This person organizes the administrative functions of the hospital, delegates duties, establishes formal meetings with staff, and provides the hospital with administrative direction (Fig. 12.1).

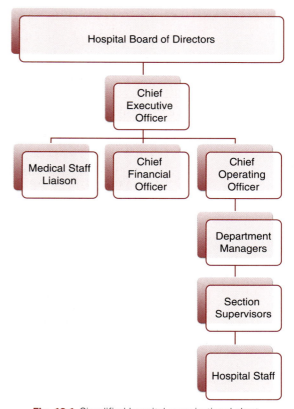

Fig. 12.1 Simplified hospital organizational chart.

Radiology Staff Activities

Most radiology departments also operate under a pyramidal administrative structure. This type of structure allows a few administrators to manage a large number of employees. Communication from the top down is usually formal so that when an order is issued from a top administrator, it is passed down to the lower levels of the pyramid without undue difficulty. However, clear and accurate communication in all directions is critical to the harmonious operation of the department.

Organizational charts and departmental **flowcharts** establish clear lines of authority, responsibility, and accountability to provide proper spans of control, create appropriate independence of operations, and define administrative record-keeping responsibilities. A plan for internal control should be implemented. This plan establishes the methods and procedures necessary to safeguard assets, monitor the accuracy and reliability of accounting data, promote managerial efficiency, and encourage adherence to managerial policy (Fig. 12.2).

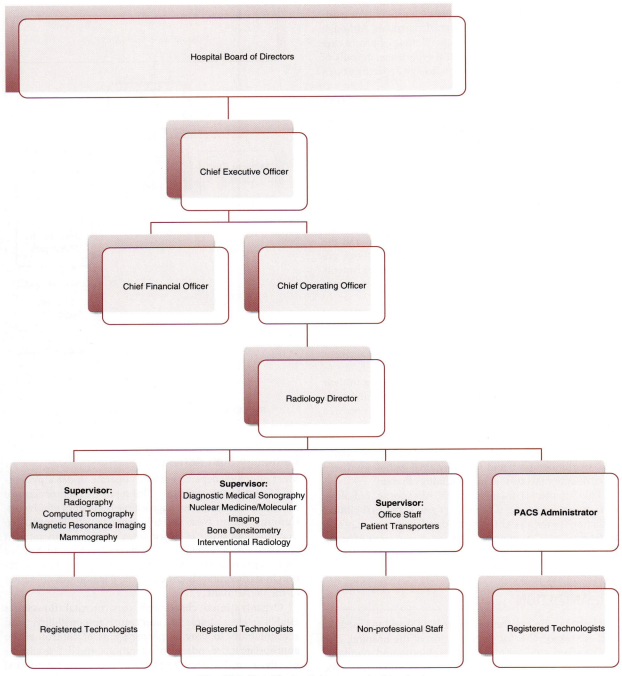

Fig. 12.2 Simplified radiology organization chart.

The ultimate objective of the diagnostic radiology department is to aid physicians in their efforts to diagnose and treat disease by providing them with timely and reliable information obtained from radiographic examinations using the least amount of radiation necessary. To ensure the reliability of this diagnostic information, careful attention must be given to the performance of every examination, beginning when the examination is ordered and continuing until the examination results have been returned to the requesting physician. This relentless attention must come from all members of the radiology staff. Diagnostic radiology services should be conveniently available to meet the needs of the patient.

The radiology management staff and radiologists have the following responsibilities:

1. Participation in medical staff activities as required
2. Establishment of an effective working relationship with the medical staff, the administration, and other departments and services
3. Development and approval of all policies and procedures for the radiology department
4. Verification of the qualifications and capabilities of all radiology staff professional and technical personnel
5. Development of comprehensive safety rules in cooperation with the hospital safety committee
6. Review and evaluation of the quality and appropriateness of radiologic services
7. Advisement of the medical staff and administration of equipment needs, modification, and utilization

POLICIES AND PROCEDURES

Developing and approving all radiology department policies and procedures is the responsibility of the radiology administrator. When this responsibility is executed thoroughly, the radiology department should function in a smooth and organized manner.

Requesting Radiology Services

Each request for radiologic examinations is reviewed for completeness of information by the radiologic technologist. Precautions regarding infection control and isolation information and detailed instructions on how to move or transport the patient should be indicated on the request form. Ensuring that these examinations are performed promptly and efficiently according to radiation safety criteria and legal codes is the responsibility of the radiology manager in conjunction with the radiologist. The radiology manager is also responsible for ensuring that other radiology-related legal codes, quality assurance, and continuing education needs are met to ensure that the patient is given the best quality care in the most effective manner.

Procedures Manual

Many radiology departments develop their own radiology information or protocol manuals and make them available to other departments, physicians, or associated institutions. These **procedures manuals** are generally designed to meet accreditation standards, state standards, and hospital codes. Many radiology departments include general instructions for patients who visit the department. The instructions may cover such subjects as appropriate gowning of the patient; transportation of the patient; precautions to be observed in the transport of very confused, ill, medicated, or feeble patients; and, when indicated, patient isolation procedures.

The manual usually includes samples of authorization forms for various radiographic studies, even if the forms are executed electronically. Because of their potential hazards, many radiographic studies require the authorization or consent of the patient before the study is performed. The manual usually includes a section of instructions about the preparation of a patient for contrast studies. This process may include the sequencing of each radiographic procedure that uses contrast agents; it may also designate the radiographic examinations that may be performed on the same day. This information is helpful to students or new personnel who are learning the policies and procedures specific to their particular area. The description of each radiographic examination covered in the manual includes the details of the procedure, as well as the preparation for the study.

A disaster drill program is implemented by the administrator of the hospital for each participating department. The manual may include a section about the disaster drill program so that it is available to all radiology personnel.

Human Resource Procedures

Even though the hospital human resources department maintains records about all hospital employees, the radiology administrator is responsible for verifying the qualifications and capabilities of all radiology staff personnel.

Staff records should contain background information that is adequate to justify the initial employment of an applicant. Applicants requiring a license or certification for employment are usually employed only after verification of an active credential. Periodic work-performance evaluations should be recorded, and employee health records should be kept on file. Subsequent health services are rendered to employees to ensure that they are physically able to perform their assigned duties and are free of active disease.

After they have been established and maintained, these written policies and practices should support optimal achievement and quality patient care. These policies should be provided to employees and discussed in their initial orientation to the department.

Safety

Safety in the health care environment for both the patient and the employee is very important. Equipment safety is a major concern in many institutions as a result of the proliferation of medical equipment and the increase in the number and complexity of diagnostic tests requested by physicians. Standards set for hospital accreditation require not only initial compliance but also—and more important—a continuing program of testing and preventive maintenance.

Electrical safety is important in the radiology department because of the high-voltage equipment used; it is also a concern of the entire hospital. Therefore an electrical safety policy is a hospital-wide program. An awareness of the use of electronic equipment in diagnostic and therapeutic patient support is essential for all personnel. Written policies and procedures about electrical safety are essential.

In the radiology department, The Joint Commission recommends that radiation safety precautions be established by a **radiation safety committee.** It is responsible for monitoring and maintaining a radiation-safe environment, in cooperation with the **hospital safety committee,** which is responsible for safety in all areas of the hospital. The recommendations of the National Council on Radiation Protection and Measurements are given as a standard that should be known and applied.

Personnel monitoring is the measuring of the radiation exposure received by personnel in the performance of their duties. This is accomplished by wearing a dosimeter, either an optically stimulated luminescence badge or a thermoluminescent dosimeter badge (Figs. 12.3 and 12.4). Dosimeter reports should be reviewed on a monthly or quarterly basis to ensure levels of exposure are at safe levels. The dosimeter reports must be posted in an appropriate area for staff access. As a student, you will also wear a dosimeter and review and initial the dosimeter report.

Radiation protection devices and accessories should be readily available. Equipment such as lead gloves, lead aprons, and radiation beam–restricting devices should be monitored on a regularly scheduled basis.

Equipment calibration and safety maintenance are a part of the function of a radiology department. The accrediting agency recommends that diagnostic and therapeutic equipment be calibrated in accordance with federal, state, and local requirements.

Rules for the safe use, removal, handling, and storage of radioactive elements and their disintegrating products should be established and enforced. In addition to rules for the radiology department staff, rules should be developed for the protection of all facility staff members who care for patients treated with these substances. All compliance procedures must be performed on a regular basis and documented.

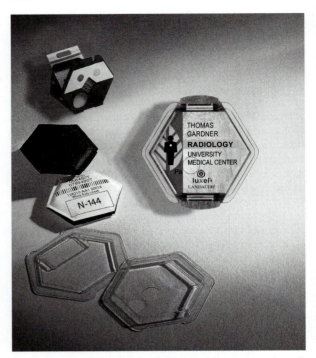

Fig. 12.3 Optically stimulated luminescence dosimeters for radiology personnel. (From Sherer M, Visconti P, Ritenour E, Haynes K: *Radiation protection in medical radiography*, ed 8, St. Louis, 2018, Elsevier.)

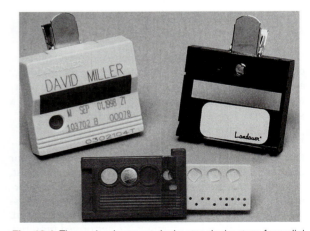

Fig. 12.4 Thermoluminescent dosimeter dosimeters for radiology personnel. (From Sherer M, Visconti P, Ritenour E, Haynes K: *Radiation protection in medical radiography*, ed 8, St. Louis, 2018, Elsevier.)

Compliance evaluations, which include the inspection and testing of x-ray units, should be performed at the recommended intervals. These tests include tabletop exposure rate measurements, half-value layer determinations, scatter radiation surveys, and accuracy checks. Measurements of the adequacy of structural shielding as required by state regulations should be assessed and documented. All tests and inspections must be documented to satisfy the record-keeping requirements for accreditation and state law.

Sanitation and Infection Control

Sanitation practices are of great concern to departments of radiology because so many patients are seen in the department daily. Radiologic technologists and staff do not spend a great deal of time with each patient, but they see a large number of patients each day. Maintaining a clean environment is essential. Rooms should be kept neat, clean, and orderly. Building and service equipment, such as air conditioning and ventilation systems, must be well maintained. Attention must be given to storage areas, waste disposal, and laundry. Sanitation practices and policies must also be a hospital-wide concern.

Infection control affects the entire hospital, as well as the radiology department (see Fig. 12.4). The accrediting body for hospitals recommends a hospital-wide infection control program. Some elements of the infection control program are mechanisms for reporting and identifying infections, maintaining records of infections among patients and personnel, and reviewing and evaluating aseptic isolation and sanitation techniques. Written policies about patient isolation procedures and control procedures relating to the hospital environment, which includes central service, housekeeping, laundry, engineering, food, and waste management, are developed for hospital-wide use.

The importance of hand washing as the number one controlling factor of infection cannot be overstated.

The Joint Commission publishes a manual addressing hospital accreditation that establishes standards for hospital services. The hospital in its entirety is viewed as responsible for overseeing, coordinating, and integrating its activities and functions. Therefore, the aggregation of rules and recommendations are integrated with standards and scoring guidelines. It is described by The Joint Commission and is based on a paradigm of integrating activities and functions.

The **Occupational Safety and Health Administration (OSHA)** is a federal agency that is concerned with safety in the workplace. The safe handling and disposal of hazardous materials is a major concern of OSHA; it establishes standards for safety in the workplace universally. These standards are mandated by law.

REIMBURSEMENT

Until the early 1970s, the primary concern of both the health care industry and the federal government was to modernize, expand, and purchase new equipment to provide the public with more and better health care. However, during the mid-1970s, the thrust of government and the health care industry changed. The high cost of health care was, in part, the cause of this change. The government responded to public pressure by imposing numerous regulations on hospitals and other health care institutions. Almost all aspects of hospital operations were reached by government regulations.

Discussion of reimbursement for health care services remains current with the ongoing debate over the advantages and disadvantages of the **Affordable Care Act**. The role of the federal government (i.e., taxpayers) in funding health care is likely to be further defined as time goes by. The Affordable Care Act will be funded, repealed, or modified in some way. What is certain is that health care services will continue to be managed in the most cost-effective manner possible.

Prospective Payment for Medicare

Prospective reimbursement is the federal government's response to the problem of skyrocketing health costs. The health care inflation rate has grown many times faster than the overall inflation rate of the United States. The principal reason that health care costs have become so inflated is that, in the past, hospitals had no real incentive to control them. Basically, the government reimbursed the hospitals for whatever kind of test or treatment was performed.

To understand how **Medicare** prospective payment became a reality, we must look back to 1965, when the federal government began offering Medicare for older adults and **Medicaid** for low-income persons and families. These programs were established with a cost-based system for reimbursing medical treatment. No incentive was provided to control costs, and this open-ended reimbursement system in effect rewarded excessive admissions and services and inefficient use of high technology.

Other factors that contributed to the rising cost of health care included the malpractice epidemic, which resulted in physicians using more tests. However, the number one costs in health care are hospital employee salaries and benefits. Therefore, in essence, all share in the rising health care costs.

The concern and public outcry over runaway health care costs led to the new system of prospective reimbursement for Medicare. Under this system, payments are limited to the set amount allocated to the specific diagnosis. Under cost-based reimbursement, a hospital could spend a dollar and be assured of getting part of it back. Under this system, a hospital has the opportunity to make a dollar by saving a dollar.

The radiology department moved from being a profit center to a cost center, and the emphasis is now on improving productivity and efficiency.

Because of the **prospective payment system**, certain medical services, including some medical imaging, have moved out of the acute care hospital and into less costly facilities. These facilities include freestanding urgent care centers, imaging centers, outreach clinics, physical rehabilitation facilities, sports medicine clinics, and various other health care entities. Hospitals are now contracting with physicians and corporations to provide services at a fixed fee.

ECONOMICS OF RADIOLOGY

Radiology, laboratory, and pharmacy are three important revenue-producing departments in a hospital. These departments help support nonrevenue areas such as administration, human resources, maintenance, and housekeeping.

A radiology department should be operated efficiently and cost effectively. It is one of the most expensive hospital departments to operate, supply, and equip. Radiologic technologists have the opportunity to make a significant difference in the cost effectiveness of the operation of the department. Several ways can be used to make this difference. Perhaps the most important one, however, is to prevent the need for repeating examinations because of technical errors, which not only reduces costs, but also prevents the patient from receiving unnecessary radiation.

Another method of reducing operating costs is to schedule examinations for maximal unit, equipment, and personnel use. Consistently practicing conservation in the use of materials and supplies throughout all areas of the department will have a considerable effect over time.

The student radiologic technologist should be aware that economics is as important in radiology as are the other aspects of the profession. Mere technical quality is of little consequence if the cost of the service makes it prohibitive for the patient. Quality patient care means caring for the patient, and this effort clearly includes the patient's financial concerns. Furthermore, Medicare reimbursement also takes into account patient satisfaction scores, so excellent patient care and patient service are of paramount importance.

Staffing

As mentioned previously, the staff of a radiology department represents an important part of a hospital's labor force and cost. On the technical side, this staff normally consists of an administrative director, shift supervisors, radiologic technologists, clerical staff, and support staff (e.g., patient transporters). The medical side consists of the radiologists, who are usually a corporation under contract with the hospital to provide their services.

The personnel required to staff an imaging department depends on departmental systems and procedures. The number and function of these employees are based on the volume and type of procedures performed. Overstaffing reduces staff use and creates increased labor costs. Having the appropriate staffing level to provide good patient care with high productivity is economically necessary.

Equipment

The radiology administrator, the hospital CEO, and the radiologists are responsible for the selection of imaging equipment. The imaging technology in a radiology department represents some of the most expensive equipment in a hospital. Costs range from tens of thousands of dollars for a **mobile (portable) unit** (i.e., an x-ray machine designed for easy movement for radiographing patients outside of the radiology department) to millions of dollars for computed tomography and magnetic resonance imaging scanners (Fig. 12.5). The selection of appropriate radiographic equipment is a complicated procedure; the department administrator must analyze how many radiographic rooms are necessary and what type of equipment is required to perform the procedures efficiently. An analysis of the types and frequency of procedures offered should be made.

Consequently, spending thousands of dollars for equipment that will not be used effectively is not economically sound. When purchasing new equipment, the availability of maintenance and repair services should be analyzed. Spending large sums of money on imaging equipment when no local maintenance services are available is senseless. Each hour and day a radiographic unit is inoperable,

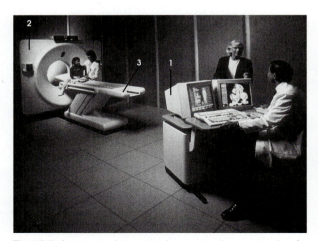

Fig. 12.5 A computed tomography scanner is an example of a very expensive yet vital component of imaging departments. Components: 1, computer and operator's console; 2, gantry; 3, patient table. (Long B, Rollins J, Smith B: *Merrill's atlas of radiographic positioning and procedures*, ed 13, St. Louis, 2016, Elsevier.)

the department and hospital lose revenue. Therefore service is one of the prime considerations in deciding what brand of equipment to purchase.

Maintenance contracts are negotiated with manufacturers before the issuance of a purchase order for the equipment to get the lowest possible contract price. After the equipment is purchased, any leverage in negotiating the maintenance contract is lost. This factor is important because the imaging equipment should have the lowest possible life-cycle cost. **Life-cycle cost** is defined as the acquisition cost of the equipment plus the cost of maintaining it through its useful life.

QUALITY ASSURANCE AND QUALITY CONTROL

The radiology administrator and the radiology management staff must maintain **quality assurance**, which is the monitoring and testing of imaging equipment and the control of variables that include personnel in the clinical setting, minimizing the unnecessary duplication of radiographic examinations, and maximizing the quality of diagnostic information. They must also review and evaluate the quality and appropriateness of radiologic services.

Quality is often defined as a degree of excellence. Everyone who enters a health care facility expects to receive the highest possible quality—or excellence—of service. The radiologic technologist plays an important role in maintaining that quality of service.

Quality assurance is a term that encompasses radiology staff, equipment, accessories, and delivery of imaging services. *Quality control* is a term referring to the hardware or equipment in radiology departments.

Every hospital radiology department has a quality assurance program, as required by law. It involves all radiology personnel in how they will perform their tasks, as well as the equipment for function and safety. Large departments may designate one person to be responsible for the program. However, most departments make all technologists responsible for quality assurance within their **scope of practice**.

Radiographic Equipment

The radiographic equipment is the first thing that most people consider as the major concern of high-quality radiographic services. In many respects, this concern is justified because radiographic equipment is indeed the most complex and potentially complicating factor in the entire pyramid. Regardless of the complexity and intricacy of the equipment, tests to identify the problem are well developed. During the course of your study, you will learn about these tests and what the results mean.

The equipment is the most likely place to begin a search for the source of a problem. This aspect is especially true when a problem persists throughout a large number of different patients and procedures. The most reliable method of attacking equipment problems is the **troubleshooting** technique. This method is similar to the process a physician uses in diagnosing a disease. First, begin by thinking of all the possible causes of the problem. Then, one by one, in order of probability, rule out causes. If this procedure does not pinpoint the cause, think of other possible causes. Although time consuming, this method will lessen the possibility of totally ignoring important facts.

Special tools allow the quality assurance technologist to check the quality of the radiographic equipment. Most of these tests are performed using a digital dosimeter to determine variances in x-ray output. In most cases, quality control testing is performed by a contracted agency external to the hospital. Medical radiation physicists play a large part in a quality control program.

Every new radiologic technology student is overwhelmed by the complexity of the equipment and the sophisticated techniques used by staff radiologic technologists. However, as a student, several steps can be taken to ensure quality, even in the early stage of your clinical education, such as making sure equipment is handled carefully and kept clean. As you spend more time in clinical education, you will soon become accustomed to using complex machines and methods to produce radiographic images. However, an important point to remember is that radiographic services are very complex and sophisticated, no matter how familiar they may become. In fact, this complexity is the primary problem in maintaining quality radiographic services in today's radiology departments.

Radiographer

Proper orientation to the equipment and procedures necessary for the operation of x-ray equipment should always be addressed first. Good quality assurance requires all users of new equipment to have a proper orientation regarding the correct usage of the equipment.

The radiographer has nearly total control over the quality of radiographic services provided, determining proper exposure technique and providing quality patient care and service. Thus, the radiographer's skill, judgment, and integrity play major roles in maintaining quality. It is vital to perform imaging examinations exactly as they are to be done, avoiding shortcuts and compromises. Proper positioning of the patient, the part to be imaged, and using exact central ray entrance and exit points are critical to optimal image quality.

A professional is competent in **positioning skills**. Simply learning the standard and routine procedures for your institution is usually not sufficient to reach this goal. To position difficult patients, you must know positioning well enough to adapt a common procedure to an unusual situation and still produce a high-quality radiograph. This task can be difficult, especially if the patient is uncooperative because of extreme pain or if the patient is unable to understand what you are attempting to do.

The best methods of overcoming these problems are (1), practicing routine procedures until you are thoroughly familiar with them and (2) paying close attention to the techniques used by staff radiologic technologists in unusual situations. Using the proper centering points, tube angles, and patient positioning are crucial.

The radiographer has total control over the selection of **exposure factors**. Imaging equipment uses automatic exposure controls and anatomically programmed radiography for many examinations (Figs. 12.6 and 12.7). However, such controls are not applicable to all radiographic situations. Many instances (e.g., during portable radiography) exist when the radiographer must select all of the exposure factors to be used for the examination. In these instances, adjustments in exposure factors must be made. Guessing is never acceptable. Working through a complex problem step by step is a scientific approach that nearly always provides an acceptable set of exposure factors (Fig. 12.8).

Patients

You will encounter a significant number of roadblocks in your efforts to achieve an optimal quality rating. Not only do your patients come in various heights, weights, and widths, with injuries and pathologies, but they also arrive for your care with various temperaments and attitudes. You will study in depth the art and science of acquiring diagnostic images; these studies will help you to solve the problem of your patients' various body sizes and conditions. The problem of your patients' psychological and emotional states, however, is one that you must constantly strive to solve. Many radiologic technologists who enjoy their work profess that solving these types of problems is the factor that makes their work interesting and rewarding. This is all a part of quality assurance.

You should learn to evaluate your patients before you begin to prepare them for examination. Treat older patients with respect, younger patients with smiles and interesting questions, extremely ill patients with gentleness, and dying patients with compassion but not pity. You will soon learn the best methods for "getting on the good side" of each of your patients. If you remember that most patients enter the radiology department with some apprehension and uncertainty, you will have a good basis for understanding how to approach their psychological and emotional problems. You must relieve their apprehensions by demonstrating that they are special to you and that you are competent in your job. You can relieve their uncertainty by explaining exactly what you are going to do before you begin the radiographic examination.

Creating Good Physical Conditions

Creating the proper physical conditions for your patients is one of the most effective methods for alleviating their apprehensions. You can accomplish this task in several ways:

1. Read the examination request to learn your patient's name and what radiographic procedure is to be performed.
2. Set up the examination room for the proper procedure by making sure the radiographic tube, table, and other

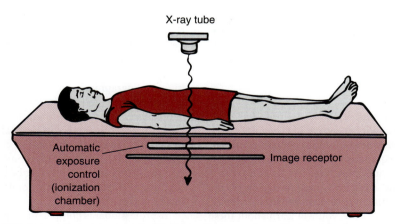

X-ray tube

Automatic exposure control (ionization chamber)

Image receptor

Fig. 12.6 Automatic exposure control is located between the patient and the image receptor.

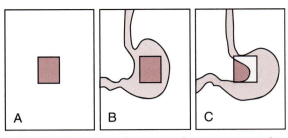

Fig. 12.7 Proper use of an automatic exposure control.

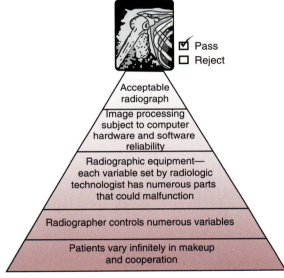

Fig. 12.8 Pyramidal radiograph.

items are in a position that facilitates moving the patient into the room and into position for the examination.

3. Explain to the patient that you are locating the exact area to be imaged; then touch gently as you position them.
4. Provide comfort items as necessary, such as sponges to assist in holding uncomfortable positions and pillows and sheets for modesty.

All of these procedures help create a cooperative and responsive patient, which in turn allows for delivery of quality patient care.

Maintaining Competency

Continuing education provides a means for professionals to keep abreast of advancements in radiologic technology. Because of the rapidly advancing nature of the profession, no individual can afford to rest securely on the knowledge received during the traditional educational program. As new ideas and techniques are introduced into the field, each person must find a way to learn and use this new knowledge. Attending professional society conferences and in-service education programs and reading current professional journal articles help radiologic technologists absorb this wealth of information.

Administrative Evaluation

A very important aspect of quality assurance focuses on staff. The radiology department administration is very interested in how staff technologists deal with patient problems. Managers might use any of the following techniques to observe the quality of patient care: observation of technologists at work, interviewing patients, and interviewing technologists. An in-service workshop on patient care or an informal discussion about dealing with patient problems often brings to light particular problems with which radiologic technologists need help.

All of these techniques help managers discover the quality of patient care services in radiology. The patient's optimal rating of the radiology department, as well as successful radiograph production, depends on meeting both the patient's psychological and physical needs.

Technologists normally have performance evaluations on an annual basis. This is an opportunity for one-on-one conversation between the supervisor and the radiographer regarding the delivery of patient care and working with fellow staff members.

Radiologist

Ultimately, the radiologist is the most important determinant of quality assurance. *The radiologist is the only person in the department who may legally make a diagnosis from a radiograph.* This statement means that, even though the radiographer is the expert in the *production* of the radiographic image, the *diagnosis* from the image is always provided by the radiologist. Consequently, the true function of the radiographer can be viewed as someone who produces images that the brain and eyes of the radiologist can form into meaningful diagnostic information.

Maintaining Personal Standards

Radiographers differ from one another in their personal acceptance limits; the image that one technologist accepts may be repeated by another. To help minimize variation in departmental acceptance limits, many departments designate one or more radiographers as quality control technologists who review images on the *picture archive and communication system.* In this manner, the supervisor's acceptance level becomes the departmental acceptance level. When these individuals have a long acquaintance with the acceptance levels of the radiologists in the department, they can effectively serve as a screening mechanism for the images the radiologists view.

Students often have two different standards of radiographic acceptability—one that they use when their clinical instructors are present and another that they use when they work on their own. A true professional must develop personal standards that do not vary, regardless of whether teachers, department managers, or anyone else is present.

An important factor is effective communication. Radiographers often encounter instances when patients refuse—as is their right—to allow repeat exposures. On occasion, a physician may need to take a patient into surgery and will not allow you to repeat an exposure. Occasionally, patients may be uncooperative, or trauma or a pathologic condition might interfere with making an acceptable radiograph. In all of these situations, explaining to the radiologist the circumstances that prohibited maintaining acceptance limits is important.

Communication is also important when obtaining medical histories from your patients. Learn to ask the correct questions of your patients. As you learn more about patient assessment, you will discover that if you can locate the precise area of pain and describe it correctly for the radiologist, you can add to the diagnostic information available for reading the radiograph. Historic information, such as the duration of the pain and its intensity, can affect the accuracy of the radiologic diagnosis. The medical history is just as important as the completeness and quality of the image produced on the radiograph.

CONCLUSION

The radiology department is a complex operation. Every member of the department needs to be aware of the responsibilities and organizational structure of the department. This awareness—coupled with the dedicated, cooperative performance of these responsibilities on the part of radiology personnel—can make patients' visits to the department as pleasant and employees' service to the department as meaningful and satisfying as possible. All imaging services must be delivered in a cost-effective manner. Medicare reimbursement is partly based on patient satisfaction scores, so delivering high-quality, empathetic care is vital for the patient and for the fiscal foundation of the department.

QUESTIONS FOR DISCUSSION AND CRITICAL THINKING

1. Discuss reasons why understanding the overall organization of a hospital and a radiology department are important to a radiographer.
2. Describe the importance of a procedures manual to a radiography student and a new radiographer hire.
3. Explain the importance of wearing a dosimeter.
4. Discuss the importance of hand washing and an infection control program.
5. Describe factors impacting the financial health of an imaging department.
6. Contrast quality control with quality assurance.
7. Describe the role of the radiographer in diagnosing a condition.

BIBLIOGRAPHY

Bushong S. *Radiologic science for technologists*. ed 11. St. Louis: Elsevier; 2017.

Carlton R. Establishing a total quality assurance program in diagnostic radiology. *Radiol Technol*. 1980; 52(1):23, 1980.

Carter D, Veale B. *Digital radiography and PACS*. ed 3. St. Louis: Elsevier; 2018.

The Joint Commission. *Accreditation manual for hospitals*. Oakbrook Terrace, IL: Author; 2018.

Long B, Rollins J, Smith B. *Merrill's atlas of radiographic positioning and procedures*. ed 13. St. Louis: Elsevier; 2016.

Morrison G. Trends in health care workplace. *Radiol Technol*. 2006; 6(77):433–435.

Papp J. *Quality management in the imaging sciences*. ed 6. St. Louis: Elsevier; 2018.

Price P. Equipment safety and risk management. *Radiol Technol*. 2004; 75(3):211.

Sherer M, Visconti P, Ritenour E, Haynes K. *Radiation protection in medical radiography*, ed 8. St. Louis, Elsevier; 2018.

Sherry C. Financial issues facing radiology executives. *Radiol Today*. 2008; 9(24):40–43.

US Department of Health and Human Services. http://www.fda.gov.

Wesolowski CE. Let's put "care" back into health care. *Radiol Manag*. 1990; 12(3):49–55.

Wilson D. World economic outlook for 2009. *Bus Perspect*. 2009; 19(4):38–45.

13

Health Professions

OBJECTIVES

On completion of this chapter, you should be able to:
- Give a historical account of how the allied health professions developed.
- Describe the role of each allied health profession discussed in this chapter.
- Discuss the importance of the health care team.

OUTLINE

KEY TERMS

allied health
cytotechnologist
dietitian
emergency medical personnel
histologic technician

health information management (HIM)
medical technologists
nurse
occupational therapist

physical therapist
physician assistant (PA)
respiratory therapist

One of the most important changes that occurred during the evolution and progression of scientific medicine in this country was the tendency of health providers to specialize. **Allied health**, which is a group of specialized, complex, and highly technical professions, grew, developed, and proliferated out of this specialization, which brought with it the need to develop efficient working relationships among the numerous medical professionals, as well as among the organizational components of health services. These relationships needed to extend beyond the health field into other areas, including science and industry. Specialization allowed health professionals to develop more complex skills and expertise in their fields.

As the population has increased and medical care has become more sophisticated, the role of allied health professions has greatly expanded. Many new professions have emerged as more duties and responsibilities once performed by physicians and dentists have shifted to allied health personnel. Allied health personnel can be trained more quickly and less expensively than physicians and dentists, who can now make better use of their time and skills.

Some of the allied health professions are well established and well known; others have just emerged and parallel the introduction of new technology. You should be aware of the tasks performed by allied health providers in your work environment and the role they play in the health care team.

This chapter discusses some health professions you may encounter in your clinical experience, but it by no means covers all of them. The US Department of Health and Human Services, a federal government department with the responsibility for providing services in health care, has identified more than 250 health-related occupations. The following descriptions introduce you to a few of these other health care team members.

EMERGENCY MEDICAL TECHNICIAN OR PARAMEDIC

Immediate care of sick and injured patients is of paramount importance, and an emergency medical technician (EMT) or paramedic is often the first person to tend to the patient's needs. **Emergency medical personnel** must have competence in the areas of prehospital care, patient transportation, patient and family counseling, providing medical care under the direction of an emergency physician, and maintaining emergency vehicles and biomedical equipment. EMTs are trained to administer life support and definitive therapy via radio communication with physicians.

Prerequisites for an EMT program include high school graduation or its equivalent. The program includes classroom and clinical work and a field internship. The paramedic credential requires a minimum of 2 years of education.

MEDICAL LABORATORY SCIENTIST (CLINICAL LABORATORY SCIENCE)

The medical laboratory scientist functions within the clinical laboratory to provide diagnostic and therapeutic information to primary caregivers. This information is generated by the medical laboratory scientist through highly precise analysis of blood and body fluids to measure and identify the constituents. Several different disciplines or specialties are within the profession of medical technology. Clinical laboratory science includes such disciplines as hematology, clinical chemistry, immunohematology (blood banking), microbiology, immunology, and molecular diagnostics.

Body fluid chemistry involves measurement of constituents such as glucose, cholesterol, blood acidity, and the various blood proteins. Hematologic analyses include counting red and white blood cells and using the microscope to identify abnormalities. Clotting abnormalities also can be identified by a variety of special tests. Medical laboratory scientists working in the blood banking discipline test donor and recipient blood to ensure compatibility of transfusion products. In the microbiology laboratory, **medical technologists** culture and analyze bacteria, fungi, parasites, and viruses to diagnose infectious diseases while also performing tests to determine the most effective therapeutic agents. Immunodiagnostic testing involves the detection of immune system products such as antibodies to determine infectious disease status, as well as protective immunity. A newly emerging discipline in medical technology involves molecular testing such as analysis of deoxyribonucleic acid (DNA).

To perform these tasks, medical laboratory scientists must apply technical skills, and they also must understand the related chemical, physical, and biologic principles necessary to ensure accurate laboratory results. The educational requirements to become a medical technologist take approximately 4 years and involve completion of chemistry, biology, math, English, and elective prerequisites after which the student attends an accredited program of medical technology to focus on both classroom and practical experiences in all the disciplines to complete a baccalaureate degree. After educational requirements are complete, the graduate is eligible to sit for one or more of the national certification examinations in medical technology. The most recognized certification as a medical technologist is offered by the American Society for Clinical Pathology, which results in the MLS (ASCP) credential.

The traditional work settings for medical technologists are in the hospital clinical laboratory or in large independent laboratories. However, many medical technologists work in other settings such as research or education or in the laboratory supply industry as technical representatives.

HISTOTECHNOLOGY

The field of histotechnology is fairly small; approximately 9000 registered histologic technicians practice in the United States. A **histologic technician** processes tissue samples from surgical autopsies and research procedures. These technicians may work in university hospitals, research centers, or private laboratories. They must be skilled in processing tissue from surgical and autopsy procedures, embedding tissue into paraffin blocks; cutting ultra-thin, paraffin-embedded tissue samples; and identifying tissue by sight and stain.

The curriculum for histologic technicians requires instruction in medical terminology, medical ethics, chemistry, anatomy, histology, and histochemistry. The program also includes clinical education in instrumentation, microscopy, and processing techniques. Programs in histotechnology are accredited by the National Accrediting Agency for Clinical Laboratory Sciences.

The educational entrance requirements to an accredited program include a high school diploma or equivalent plus

1 year of supervised training in a qualified pathology laboratory or graduation from an accredited program of histologic technique. A college background in chemistry, biology, and mathematics may be helpful. Certification as a histologic technician is through examination by the Board of Registry of Medical Technologists and has been given the designation HT (ASCP).

CYTOTECHNOLOGY

Cytotechnology is a growing field in the allied health sciences. It involves the microscopic study of cells that have been exfoliated or abraded from body tissues to reveal abnormalities that could implicate cancer. With the help of cytotechnology, the physician is often able to diagnose and treat cancer before symptoms occur or before it can be detected by other methods.

Cytotechnology originated as a method of detecting malignant and premalignant lesions in the female genital tract. This test, which is commonly known as the Pap smear, was named after Dr. George Papanicolaou, the test's developer. Today cytotechnology has expanded to include cancer detection in all body areas, as well as the detection of other disease processes and genetic disorders.

A **cytotechnologist** works with pathologists in hospital laboratories, universities, and private laboratories and perform various specialized techniques used in the collection, preparation, and staining of cell samples; therefore, cytotechnology requires an extensive knowledge of anatomy, physiology, and the diseases of cells, tissues, and organ systems to interpret cell morphology.

Prerequisites for entering cytology programs are 4 years in an accredited college or university with an area of concentration in biologic sciences, certification as a registered medical laboratory scientist, or a baccalaureate degree from an accredited college or university with an emphasis in biology. The clinical program follows. Graduates of an accredited program are certified through the American Society of Clinical Pathologists and are recognized as CT (ASCP) cytotechnologists.

HEALTH INFORMATION MANAGEMENT

The work of **health information management (HIM)** personnel encompasses a wide variety of tasks, including planning, organizing, and directing the activities of the HIM department; preparing, maintaining, and analyzing records and reports of patient illnesses; and assisting the medical staff in research studies and evaluation of the quality of medical care. Communication skills are critical (Fig. 13.1). They provide coded data on diagnoses and procedures for reimbursement of health care encounters. HIM

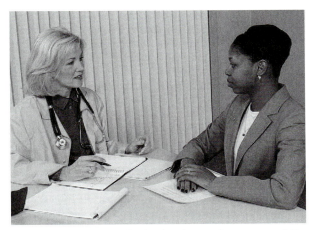

Fig. 13.1 Clear communication is a key to the success of the health information management professional. (From Pagliarulo MA: *Introduction to physical therapy*, ed 5, St. Louis, 2016, Elsevier.)

personnel also develop secondary records (e.g., disease and operations indexes and statistics for medical staff and hospital administration) and maintain the privacy and security of confidential patient information. In addition, HIM personnel are involved in the movement by health care facilities to the electronic medical record.

The professional education program includes anatomy and physiology, medical terminology, health information science, current ICD (International Statistical Classification of Diseases and Related Health Problems) coding, statistics, law, health information technology and systems, fundamentals of medical science, and organization and administration of health care facilities.

NUTRITION AND DIETETICS

A nutritionist or **dietitian** may work in a department of public health performing patient education and counseling or in a hospital operating food service, planning modified menus and therapeutic diets, and counseling patients. He or she may also work in a nursing home as a dietary consultant in both therapeutic and administrative functions or with a food-processing company aiding in the testing of food products.

A dietetics program includes a 4-year baccalaureate program with the addition of a dietetic internship. The internship may be completed concurrently with the undergraduate program, or a year's dietetic internship may be taken at an approved hospital, medical center, or commercial institution. The curriculum covers a broad range of topics, including nutrition and disease, maternal and child nutrition, and nutrition and aging. Admission to the American Dietetic Association requires an advanced degree or a dietetic traineeship. Dietitians and nutritionists are accredited by the American Dietetic Association, which was founded in 1917. Continuing education is mandatory, and each member must complete 75 continuing education hours over a period of 5 years.

PHYSICAL THERAPY

A **physical therapist** performs therapeutic procedures that include exercise for increasing strength, endurance, coordination, and range of motion (Fig. 13.2). The physical therapist works with a team of personnel—as do other health care providers—including physicians, other health specialists, and members of the lay community. Physical therapists are mainly concerned with the restoration of function and the prevention of disability after disease, injury, or the loss of a body part; in some instances, this circumstance requires the physical therapist to spend a considerable amount of time with the patient.

The minimal educational requirement is the Doctor of Physical Therapy (DPT) degree. Physical therapists who wish to specialize in a specific area may seek advanced knowledge or skills or both in clinical practice, education, management, research, or any combination.

In addition to programs that prepare professional physical therapists, some universities and community colleges offer accredited 2-year educational programs for physical therapist assistants (PTAs). PTAs are skilled technical health care workers who, under the supervision of physical therapists, assist in patients' treatment programs.

Continuing education and professional growth are encouraged in the physical therapy profession, and the curriculum is designed so that students recognize their responsibilities to expand and improve their professional knowledge and skills and to foster continuing improvement in the delivery of health care.

OCCUPATIONAL THERAPY

Occupational therapy arose during World Wars I and II, when occupational therapists were sent to Europe out of

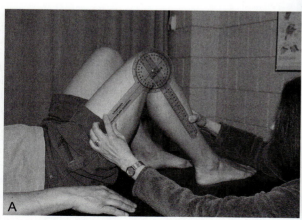
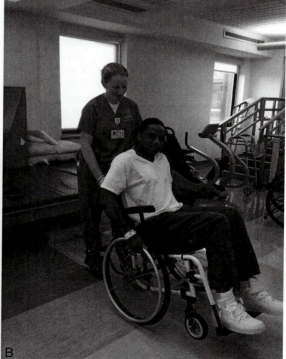

Fig. 13.2 A and **B,** Physical therapists perform key assessment and treatment for patients with physical compromises. (Part A, From Davis N, LaCour M: *Foundations of health information management*, ed 4, St. Louis, 2017, Elsevier; part B, from Pagliarulo MA: *Introduction to physical therapy*, ed 5, St. Louis, 2016, Elsevier.)

a need for advanced rehabilitation of wounded service-men. The profession has continued to become important to the promotion of health in physical, emotional, and social abilities. An **occupational therapist** evaluates the psychosocial and physical needs and capabilities of an individual, develops a treatment program and determines the necessary therapeutic activities and procedures to make the treatment program effective. Through occupational therapy, the patient's motor functions are enhanced, and psychological, social, and economic adjustments are promoted. Occupational therapists often work with patients who are regaining daily living skills with the use of artificial limbs and special equipment. They also provide instruction in activities of daily living and the use of assistive devices (Fig. 13.3).

To become certified, an occupational therapy student must fulfill the baccalaureate or master's degree requirements of an accredited program and the affiliated university or college. The program includes human sciences, human development processes, specific life tasks and activities, theory and application of occupational therapy, and field experience.

RESPIRATORY THERAPIST (RESPIRATORY CARE PRACTITIONER)

A **respiratory therapist** is an integral part of the health care team. A registered respiratory therapist (RRT) administers therapy through various procedures, such as aerosol therapy, postural drainage, and airway management, and conducts pulmonary function testing (Fig. 13.4). An RRT also responds to respiratory and cardiac emergencies and administers drugs that act in the cardiopulmonary tract.

A respiratory therapy student may attend a 24-month community college program or a 4-year baccalaureate program. Studies include anatomy and physiology, pharmacology, pathology, chemistry, technical theory, and clinical practice. The RRT examination can be taken by graduates of an accredited therapist school, and some states also require licensure examinations.

PHYSICIAN ASSISTANT

A registered **physician assistant (PA)** performs tasks that are usually conducted by the physician but that do not

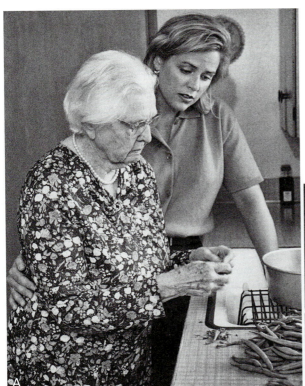
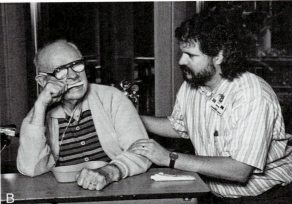

Fig. 13.3 A and **B,** Occupational therapists teach patients the daily activities of life after a stroke or other disability. (From Lohman HL, Byers-Connon S, Padilla RL: *Occupational therapy with elders: strategies for the COTA*, ed 4, St. Louis, 2019, Elsevier.)

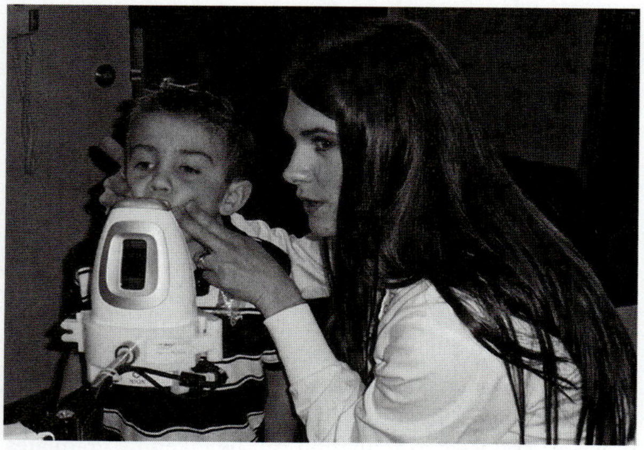

Fig. 13.4 A and **B,** Respiratory care practitioners perform vital diagnostic and therapeutic procedures. (From Walsh BK: *Neonatal and pediatric respiratory care*, ed 4, St. Louis, 2015, Elsevier.)

require such a level of expertise. These tasks include taking patient histories and performing physical examinations, follow-up care, patient teaching, counseling, and, in certain cases, diagnosis, therapy, and preventive medicine.

Prerequisites include completion of a baccalaureate degree and an additional 2+ years of PA education. Certification is through the National Commission on Certification of Physician Assistants.

NURSING

The nursing profession is the largest, oldest, and most readily identified of the health professions besides that of the physician. A **nurse** has around-the-clock contact with patients and must provide the physical and emotional support a patient needs because of illness or disability. The nurse often teaches patients and their families about illness and therapy, thereby alleviating many of their anxieties.

Registered nurses make observations and assessments that are useful to other staff members, take patient histories, give physical examinations, and administer prescribed treatments.

A nursing student can consider two routes for becoming a registered nurse. The associate degree program involves 2 years at a community college, technical institute, or university with course work in basic physical, biologic, and social sciences, humanities, and nursing. The baccalaureate program usually involves 4 academic years, and the graduate from this program most often receives a bachelor of science in nursing (BSN). Course work includes anatomy and physiology, biology, physical and social sciences, nursing, and humanities.

To become a registered nurse, the student must graduate from an approved nursing program, pass the state board

examination, and meet individual state requirements for licensure.

An advanced practice nurse (APN) must have advanced nursing skills, which usually include a master of arts or master of science in nursing. The practitioner often establishes private practice and offers services in health teaching, assessment, and physical care. An APN often has close contact with a physician for patient referral and follow-up.

The nurse anesthetist must complete an advanced program to administer anesthesia to surgery and obstetrics patients. The nurse midwife must be certified or have a master of arts in midwifery. Critical care nursing has a core curriculum of advanced specialized study and a critical care registry examination.

Nursing, as in radiologic technology, has multiple specialized functions that stimulate the growth of separate educational programs, professional organizations, and qualifying examinations and procedures.

TEAM APPROACH TO HEALTH CARE

Of all of the organizations of the health care system, the hospital is perhaps the most complex. Hospitals provide for inpatient and outpatient services of treatment and diagnosis, and many subdivisions of medical care are found within these broad functions. Hospitals must also provide professional and technical in-service education to ensure that personnel are kept abreast of new developments within their fields. Research is another important aspect of hospital care because the concentration of patients provides a database for investigation. Another function with which hospitals are involved is the prevention of disease, and this area is being given high priority in some areas, for example, isolating patients with contagious diseases.

Obviously, a hospital that is attempting to provide these services must have individuals with many diverse and highly technical skills. Equally obvious is that these individuals must work together if the goals of the health care facility are to heal the sick and to provide measures for preventive treatment. The reasons mentioned are why the team approach to health care warrants special attention.

A team can be more than the sum of its parts, just as a clock is more than the sum of its parts. The clock's function is to indicate the time, and each of its parts is precisely tooled to work in concert with the other parts to achieve this objective; so, too, must the individuals who make up the health care team work together to achieve the mission or objectives of the hospital.

Three conditions are basic to the team's ability to work together successfully. First, a clear understanding must exist of the hospital mission by all members of the team. Second, a defined purpose must exist for each technical or professional role as it relates to the mission. Third, the care provided by the team needs to be of the highest possible quality. When these three conditions exist, the team's success is ensured.

CONCLUSION

More people in the United States are engaged in health care than in any other occupation. Many factors have contributed to the establishment and rapid growth of new health occupations. Although radiologic technologists do not deal with members of all of these occupations directly, you must recognize the valuable contributions made by your colleagues on the health care team.

Specialization is a fact of life within the radiology department as much as it is in other segments of medicine. Chapter 16 provides a detailed exploration of some of the specializations available to radiologic technologists.

QUESTIONS FOR DISCUSSION AND CRITICAL THINKING

1. Discuss ways in which radiographers interact with other health care professions.
2. Compare the patient care responsibilities of the professions described in this chapter.
3. Describe the impact on patient care of the health care team working together.
4. Discuss how each profession depends on the others to provide diagnosis and treatment.

BIBLIOGRAPHY

Accreditation Review Commission on Education for the Physician Assistant. Available at http://www.arc-pa.org.
American Association of Nurse Practitioners. Available at http://www.aanp.org.
American Occupational Therapy Association. Available at http://www.aota.org.
American Physical Therapy Association. Available at http://www.apta.org.
American Society for Clinical Pathology. Available at http://www.ascp.org.

Commission on Accreditation for Respiratory Care. Available at http://www.coarc.org.
Bowman E. *Professor, Department of Health Informatics and Information Management.* Memphis, TN: University of Tennessee Health Science Center; February 2009.
Harris EL, Young P, McElveny E, et al. *The shadowmakers: a history of radiologic technology.* Albuquerque, NM: American Society of Radiologic Technologists; 1995.
Horn ML, MS RDH. University of Tennessee Health Science Center, consultant; 2009.
World Health Organization. Available at http://www.who.int/.

PART III

Growing With the Profession

14

The American Registry of Radiologic Technologists

OBJECTIVES

On completion of this chapter, you should be able to:
- Discuss the history of the American Registry of Radiologic Technologists (ARRT).
- List the professions ARRT certifies.
- Explain how test results are reported.
- Differentiate between the ARRT Rules of Ethics and the ARRT Code of Ethics.
- Explain what is meant by a continuing education (CE) biennium.
- Describe how to document proof of participation in CE.
- Identify alternative means of meeting CE requirements.
- Understand the implications of noncompliance with CE requirements.
- List sources of obtaining CE credits.

OUTLINE

KEY TERMS

academic courses
American College of Radiology (ACR)
American Registry of Radiologic Technologists (ARRT)
American Society of Radiologic Technologists (ASRT)
biennial

category A
certification
continuing education (CE) credit
continuing qualifications requirement (CQR)
in-service education
license

Radiological Society of North America (RSNA)
recognized continuing education evaluation mechanism (RCEEM)
Registered Technologist
registration
scaled scores

Certification and **registration** with the **American Registry of Radiologic Technologists (ARRT)** is the internationally recognized standard of the profession. The ARRT is recognized as the gold standard for certification in medical imaging radiation therapy. The symbol (ARRT®) has been registered with the United States Patent and Trademark

Office as the exclusive property of the ARRT, and it has become the passport to ethical employment in hospitals and clinics within English-speaking countries. Certification by the ARRT is accepted by all states with licensure laws for state licensing purposes.

The top five categories and numbers of certificates in each are:

Radiography: more than 320,000
Computed tomography (CT): more than 70,000
Mammography: nearly 50,000
Magnetic resonance imaging (MRI): more than 36,000
Radiation therapy: more than 21,000

In total, there are more than 500,000 certificates held by nearly 350,000 professionals who are qualified to work in these fields.

HISTORY OF THE AMERICAN REGISTRY OF RADIOLOGIC TECHNOLOGISTS

In 1920, four members of the **Radiological Society of North America (RSNA)** presented a plan to their organization for the certification of operators of x-ray equipment. Working together with the American Roentgen Ray Society, these two organizations established operation of the ARRT in 1922. That year, 89 certifications were given, the first of which was presented to Sister M. Beatrice Merrigan of Oklahoma City.

Also during this early period, the technicians (as technologists were then called) themselves formed the AART, which later became the American Society of X-Ray Technicians (ASXT). In April 1926, the organization voted to accept only registered technicians as members. In 1936, a joint sponsorship between the RSNA and the ASXT was established, with the ARRT incorporated as a separate body. Sponsorship again changed in 1943, when the RSNA transferred its co-sponsorship to the ACR. The ASXT continued as the other sponsor of the ARRT. At approximately the same time, the Council on Medical Education and Hospitals of the American Medical Association began to establish guidelines for x-ray courses; this effort helped to ensure quality education for students nationwide.

In 1960, work began on programs to educate and certify people in the specialties of radiation therapy and nuclear medicine technology. The first examinations for nuclear medicine were given in 1963, and the ones for radiation therapy were first given in 1964. Also in 1960, the ARRT moved to Minneapolis, Minnesota. In August 1989, the ARRT moved into its new headquarters at 1255 Northland Drive in St. Paul, Minnesota.

Persons certified by the ARRT can look back on a gratifying process of growth and acceptance: growth in professional competence and acceptance by medical, civil, and governmental organizations as the single authoritative source of qualified personnel in the disciplines the ARRT serves. The ARRT has indeed come a long way from the first Board of Registry, in which the board members personally administered their 20-question certification examination, to the present ARRT. Today's ARRT includes governance by a board of trustees and a full-time salaried staff. Primary pathway examinations are available in radiography, nuclear medicine technology, radiation therapy, MRI, and sonography. Post-primary pathway examinations are available in cardiac interventional technology (CI), vascular interventional technology (VI), mammography (M), CT, MRI, bone densitometry (BD), sonography (S), vascular sonography (VS), and breast sonography (BS). An examination is also available for radiologist assistant (RRA).

ORGANIZATION

The ARRT is governed by a board of trustees that is composed of nine members. Five trustees are registered radiologic technologists appointed by the ASRT, and four are physicians appointed by the **American College of Radiology (ACR)**. Trustees are appointed to serve 4-year terms. Meetings of the board are held semiannually, although additional meetings can be held if circumstances require. Trustees serve without compensation, but meeting expenses are reimbursed. The board is served by a full-time salaried staff who conduct the routine business of the board at the ARRT's office in St. Paul, Minnesota. The board is also served by consultants in all disciplines to which the ARRT administers examinations. These consultants provide subject expertise for the development of test questions and examinations.

Communication

Numerous publications are available on the ARRT website (www.arrt.org), including *Stories of Quality Patient Care* and *ARRT News Feed*. The handbooks for both primary and postprimary pathways are also located there.

The website also provides a mechanism to verify technologists' credentials and a link to the list of technologists who have been sanctioned.

Beginning as a student, it is wise to become familiar with www.arrt.org and to check it regularly. This is the primary method of communication between the ARRT and students and technologists.

EXAMINATION PROCEDURES

General Qualifications

Candidates must be of good moral character. Generally, conviction of either a felony or a misdemeanor indicates a lack of good moral character for ARRT purposes. Persons who have been convicted of a crime may be eligible for testing and registration after documentation has been reviewed by the Ethics Committee of the ARRT. Be sure to determine if the Ethics Review Preapplication at www.arrt.org is a route to pursue.

Educational Requirements

Candidates must have successfully completed a program of formal education and possess at least an associate degree from an institution that is accredited by a mechanism acceptable to the ARRT.

Competency Requirements

Applicants for ARRT primary pathway certification must demonstrate competency in didactic course work and, at minimum, an ARRT-specified list of clinical procedures. Most programs include additional required clinical competencies.

Application Process

During the final semester of the program, the student may apply to take the ARRT exam. In most cases, the program director will go over the application and the requirements. The application, along with the required fee, is mailed by the student to the ARRT.

The ARRT mails a Candidate Status Report to the candidate after the application is processed and testing eligibility has been determined. The Candidate Status Report contains candidate identification information, the six-digit ARRT identification number, and instructions regarding scheduling the examination.

The program director is required to verify you have completed the program at the appropriate time.

Registry Examinations

The authority and responsibility for the construction of examinations for national registration in radiologic technology have resided with the ARRT board of trustees since 1922. In the early days, the trustees set up the test specifications, wrote all test items, and administered the examinations entirely without outside help. The construction of present-day ARRT examinations is actually a combined effort of the board, its staff, and carefully selected examination committee members and item writers. The board approves the specifications for each test, including the format and item writing style. Test questions are carefully written, reviewed, and revised. Volunteer technologists and radiologists take samples of the test to verify the relevancy and difficulty level of the questions.

The examinations consist of questions using various formats. Test question formats may include multiple choice, combined response, negatively worded, select multiple, illustration, hot area (exhibits), sorted list, and video. The questions are all designed to measure the examinee's abilities to apply current knowledge in radiologic technology. See the ARRT website for examples of each type of question format.

The examinations contain 200 scored questions on the primary pathway examinations (except sonography, which has 360 questions). In addition to the scored questions, up to 20 additional pilot questions may be included that do not count toward the examinee's scores. The pilot questions are included to collect data for future use of the questions. The examinations are objective tests that cover knowledge, understanding, and application of radiologic technology practices and principles. All examinations are administered by computer at test centers under contract with the ARRT.

The test experience itself includes taking a tutorial to learn how to use the testing software. This is important to complete before beginning the exam. This does not count against the time allotted to complete the exam. Because the copyright for the examinations in radiologic technology is owned by the ARRT, the candidate is required to agree to not share test questions with anyone in any form. Two minutes is allotted to complete this agreement.

The test then begins, with questions from the various content categories being asked at random. Questions are asked over all the major topic areas learned in your program. Visit www.arrt.org for the specific test specifications in effect at the time you are in the program.

It is important to abide by all rules of the testing center, including raising your hand to ask permission to use the restroom or to leave at the completion of the exam. After you complete the exam, a questionnaire will be provided so you can give feedback on the test and testing experience.

Score Report

A preliminary score is provided on the computer screen at the test center on completion of the examination. Approximately 2 to 3 weeks after the test date, the ARRT mails score reports to all examinees. Examination results are not given over the telephone.

Scores are reported as **scaled scores**. Scaling is the process by which examinees of comparable ability who are taking different versions of the examination can be given the same reported score. Passing or failing is determined by the examinee's total score, but the total score is reported as a scaled score. The scaled score does not equal the number of questions answered correctly or the percentage of the questions answered correctly. Total scores for all examinees are converted to a score scale ranging from 1 to 99, with a scaled score of 75 defined as passing. The number of correct answers necessary to achieve a scaled score of 75 is based on the ARRT's judgment regarding what level of performance constitutes a minimal passing score and the examination of the actual scores and historical data available.

Although section scores are reported, they are not used in determining whether an examinee passes or fails but rather to provide data to the examinee that may be useful for self-evaluation purposes. The section scores are reported on a scale that ranges from 0 to 10. Again, these section scores are advisory only.

A passing score does not constitute certification unless all other requirements are also satisfied.

CERTIFICATION IN RADIOLOGIC TECHNOLOGY

Applicants for certification must agree to abide by the ARRT Rules and Regulations and the ARRT Standards of Ethics. The Standards of Ethics include the Code of Ethics and Rules of Ethics. The Code of Ethics describe what radiologic technologists aspire to be as professionals. The Rules of Ethics are enforceable rules.

To applicants who have passed the examination and are otherwise eligible, certification is issued to confer on the applicant the right to use the title **Registered Technologist** and its abbreviation, RT(ARRT), in connection with her or his name so long as the registration of the certificate is in effect. Technologists certified by the ARRT are advised to designate by the initial of their specialty of certification following the RT and to use the symbol (ARRT) in connection with RT to avoid confusion with certification from any other source. Individuals who have successfully passed examinations should use the appropriate credentials pertaining to the specific examination, such as R, N, T, CV, M, CT, MR, S, BD, VS, CI, VI, and BS.

Pocket credentials and a certificate of registration are included when the ARRT mails or emails the score report to the successful candidates. The certificate at time of issue is valid through the individual's next birth month. The certificate can be renewed from year to year on application and payment of the renewal fee as fixed by the board of trustees as long as the applicant remains qualified and meets continuing education (CE) requirements. Registrants are sent renewal applications according to their month of birth.

Continuing Education Requirements

Most graduate technologists soon realize that, although they have ended their formal education, they are at the beginning of what will prove to be a lifetime of learning.

Education presents itself in many forms. Day-to-day living provides many learning experiences that cause us to grow. Even when functioning within the specifics of a job description, we are exposed to new experiences and questions to which our education has not provided answers.

A formal educational program cannot possibly answer all questions or incorporate all potential experiences.

Understanding the ever-changing needs of radiologic technologists, the profession has established mandatory CE requirements to:
- Bridge the gap between entry-level formal education and advanced practice needs.
- Prevent professional obsolescence.
- Assure the public, our primary customers, that all technologists maintain competence.
- Demonstrate accountability to peers, physicians, health care facilities and the public.
- Advance the profession through continuous growth of all technologists working in the field.
- Provide advanced growth opportunities for technologists through advanced preparation.
- Reinforce the professional code of ethics for all practicing professionals.

Requirements

Although registered technologists must renew their ARRT registrations annually, mandatory CE requirements and documentation that the required credits have been obtained, are required on a **biennial** (2-year) basis.

The newly ARRT registered technologist will have to begin accumulating CE credits on the first day of the next birth month after becoming certified. For example, a technologist certified in March with a birth date of September 20 needs to begin acquiring CE credits on September 1. This date is the starting date of the technologist's first biennium. The biennium will extend to August 31, 2 years later, when all required credits must be completed.

A **continuing education (CE) credit** is a unit of measurement for CE activities. Each credit is based on a 50-minute contact hour.

Obtaining the required number of CE credits necessary to renew registration with the ARRT is easy if the following factors are remembered:
1. Attending, obtaining, and maintaining documentation of attendance and participation for each CE activity is solely the technologist's responsibility. This responsibility may not be delegated to anyone or any institution or organization.
2. Twenty-four credits are required during each 24-month biennium.
3. All 24 CE credits must be identified as **category A** or category A+. These activities have received approval *before* the activity attendance by a **recognized continuing education evaluation mechanism (RCEEM)**. The program listing of the CE event will indicate compliance with this requirement.

4. Credits must be educational activities relevant to the radiologic sciences or patient care.
5. The same CE activity may not be used more than once in a biennium, and CE credits for such activities as directed readings, home study courses, or Internet activities may only be used once and never repeated.

Meeting the Requirements

Typically, the most cost-effective and beneficial methods are provided by the professional societies, such as the ASRT and state or local affiliate societies. The primary purpose of these organizations is to provide for the CE needs of the professionals they represent.

Why is this the most cost-effective method? Any money spent in this way goes directly into the profession itself. Similar to a *not-for-profit* hospital, all proceeds must be used by the organization to help keep it viable. Therefore any money spent by a technologist to obtain CE from a professional society serves two purposes. The first purpose is the knowledge gained by the attendee. Second, monies spent are used by the society to help move the profession forward.

In-service education can used to obtain CE credits. These programs are developed within the institution where the technologist is employed. This type of CE may be used to address problems that affect the specific group's daily operation. For example, if repeats examinations are high within the department, an analysis may provide information with which to develop an in-service program. Remember that the program must receive approval by a RCEEM to receive CE credit.

Looking within the radiology realm is not always necessary. Patient care issues, phlebotomy, vital signs, and other basic services performed are appropriate expansions of the technologist's scope of practice and benefit the patients for which they are responsible.

Seminars by which multiple credits may be obtained are obviously faster than any single credit mechanism. Also, a method of obtaining many credits is **academic courses**. Credits are accumulated at the successful completion of the course based on a formula used by the ARRT. See the website for current information. CE should provide the technologist with new opportunities and knowledge. What better way to accomplish this task than to focus these CE efforts toward obtaining an advanced degree? Technologists are strongly encouraged to consider using this academic means of CE credit compliance.

Other sources include webinars and *directed readings* provided in professional journals, both of which can be completed at home. Although these are convenient methods of obtaining CE credits, they lack the immediacy and networking of a CE seminar or conference.

ALTERNATIVE MEANS TO MEET REQUIREMENTS

The 24-credit requirement may also be fulfilled in two other ways, as long as these alternative methods are *completed* within the individual's biennium. These methods do not require prior approval of a RCEEM:

1. A radiologic technologist may decide to continue his or her education after certification and registration in a primary discipline. The technologist may choose to enroll in an additional primary or postprimary discipline. This education will be considered to have met the CE requirements for the biennium. **NOTE:** *The additional education must be completed, and the certification examination must have been taken and passed before the end of the individual's biennium.*
2. Academic courses taken from an *accredited* postsecondary educational institution (college or university). The course must be relevant to the radiologic sciences or patient care. Relevant courses may be in:
   Biologic sciences
   Physical sciences
   Radiologic sciences
   Health and medical sciences
   Social sciences
   Communication (verbal and written)
   Mathematics
   Computers
   Management
   Education methodology

Using either option 1 or 2 above, it is vital to contact the ARRT ahead of time to verify the activity will count towards the CE requirement.

Renewal of Registration

The reminder of renewal will arrive the month before the birth month. When completing the ARRT online renewal, the technologist is asked to list the educational or learning activities completed during the biennium. Actual documentation should not accompany the renewal form. ARRT verification is performed by random sample, meaning that the ARRT will request documentation from only some of the renewing registrants. A technologist may never, may periodically, or may biennially be requested to provide documentation of CE participation. The technologist is held responsible for maintaining the necessary documentation.

Technologists employed in licensing states should check the requirements outlined by their state law. Also, technologists who function in specific modalities (e.g., mammography) may have additional federal requirements. Finally, persons certified as Registered Radiologist Assistants have requirements beyond those of the registered technologist.

Continuing Education Documentation

Proof of CE participation must be maintained by the registered technologist. Some ARRT-approved organizations, such as the **American Society of Radiologic Technologists (ASRT)**, track CE credits for their members. ASRT members may submit their CE certificates using the ASRT smartphone app. However, the technologist remains responsible for tracking and maintaining documentation. If the approved tracking organization makes an error, the ARRT will not accept this circumstance as an excuse for the lack of documentation on the part of the technologist or registrant.

The sponsor of each CE program in which a technologist participates during his or her biennium should provide documentation of attendance or participation. This documentation *must* have the following:

1. Date or dates of attendance
2. The topic or subject title
3. Content of the educational opportunity
4. Number of (50- or 60-minute) contact hours
5. Name of speaker or presenter
6. Name and signature of sponsor or authorized representative
7. The RCEEM-approved reference number, if applicable

NONCOMPLIANCE WITH CONTINUING EDUCATION REQUIREMENTS

Any technologist applying for renewal who has not obtained the necessary CE credits during their biennium or whose CE reporting form is incomplete is considered on CE probation. These individuals receive a registration card with the probation status shown.

Probation status is granted for only 6 months of the next biennium. If compliance does not occur during that 6 months, the individual is considered no longer registered by the ARRT. Applicable fees may be obtained by checking the ARRT's website (www.arrt.org).

NONRENEWAL OF REGISTRATION

As previously mentioned, potential and current employers, as well as state licensing agencies, may check the ARRT website to verify the current status of a technologist. If the technologist has not renewed registration, it indicates that the individual in question is not registered by the ARRT.

Registration reinstatement may be requested by a delinquent technologist who is subject to compliance with CE requirements. All other ARRT rules and regulations in effect at the time must be followed.

Technologists should maintain current registration with the ARRT even if they are not currently functioning within the profession. If registration is allowed to lapse beyond the individual's biennium, no reinstatement is allowed without reexamination in one of the primary disciplines.

Continuing Qualifications Requirement

The ARRT, along with numerous other health professions, has created time-limited certificates. ARRT credentials are limited to 10 years. At that time, technologists must undergo a self-assessment to determine their level of knowledge and whether they have kept up with changes and advances in the field. To accomplish this goal, **Continuing Qualifications Requirement (CQR)** was created. It applies to all credentials earned after January 1, 2011.

Technologists are contacted 3 years before the 10-year anniversary. This gives them 3 years to complete the process. CQR begins with a Structured Self-Assessment, similar to a test but only used to determine areas where CE may be needed. The self-assessment cannot be failed.

The results of the self-assessment will determine in what areas, if any, prescribed CE activities must be completed. If prescribed, the CE activities will count toward the biennium CE requirement. The technologist has 3 years in which to complete the prescribed CE.

LICENSURE REQUIREMENTS

Most states in this country require technologists to be licensed by that state. The term **license** means that legal permission has been granted by a state allowing an individual to function as a technologist and administer ionizing radiation to human beings. Technologists must take the time necessary to familiarize themselves with all national and state requirements. By not doing so, they may seriously jeopardize their ability to work in their chosen profession.

The technologist must also learn whether separate mandatory CE requirements for license renewal exist within the state of employment. Typically, the same CE credits may be used for both the ARRT and the state. However, this use should never be assumed to be accurate. Knowing when CE credits must be obtained, the number required, the acceptable types of CE, and any difference in renewal periods is the responsibility of the technologist.

CONCLUSION

The ARRT is the second largest certifying agency in the health professions, second in total numbers only to nursing. The mission of the ARRT focuses on quality patient care in imaging, interventional procedures, and radiation therapy. It accomplishes this through testing, certification, and strict adherence to high ethical standards. To ensure that registrants remain qualified, CE is a requirement. To ensure that registrants remain current, CQR is a requirement.

More than 100 years since the discovery of x-rays, we know we have only scratched the surface of our continually growing field. With the need for mandatory CE, more technologists are participating in the profession's forward movement. By all technologists committing to personal growth, we guarantee future generations of radiologic technologists will have new and even more exciting horizons to explore.

QUESTIONS FOR DISCUSSION AND CRITICAL THINKING

1. Visit the ARRT's website (www.arrt.org) and list all the modalities covered by ARRT certification. Discuss its role in the profession.
2. Discuss the general qualifications and educational requirements for applying to take the ARRT exam.
3. Visit www.arrt.org and discuss the content specifications for the radiography examination.
4. Compare the continuing education requirement with the continuing qualifications requirement.
5. Discuss the importance of keeping accurate continuing education records.
6. Explain the difference between ARRT certification and state licensure.
7. Discuss the formation, history, and evolution of the ARRT.

BIBLIOGRAPHY

American Registry of Radiologic Technologists: www.arrt.org
Gurley LT. Educational void. *Appl Radiol.* 1988; 17(11).

Harris EL, Young P, McElveny C, et al. *The shadowmakers: a history of radiologic technology.* Albuquerque, NM: American Society of Radiologic Technologists; 1995.

15

Professional Associations

OBJECTIVES

On completion of this chapter, you should be able to:

- Explain the primary mission of the American Society of Radiologic Technologists.
- Explain the purpose of the Association of Collegiate Educators in Radiologic Technology and the Association of Educators in Imaging and Radiologic Sciences.
- List other organizations to which technologists may belong.
- Explain how membership in a professional organization will benefit your personal practice of radiologic technology.
- List the organizations to which your instructors belong.
- List the many activities provided by the organizations described in this chapter by visiting each of their websites.

OUTLINE

The American Society of Radiologic Technologists: An Association for all Radiologic Science Professionals
Practice Standards for Medical Imaging and Radiation Therapy
Socioeconomics
Legislation

State and Local Affiliates
Educators
Radiology Managers and Supervisors
Other Technologist Organizations
Radiologist and Physicist Organizations
Conclusion

KEY TERMS

AHRA: The Association for Medical Imaging Management
American Society of Radiologic Technologists (ARRT)

Association of Collegiate Educators in Radiologic Technology (ACERT)

Association of Educators in Imaging and Radiologic Sciences (AEIRS)

As the field of radiologic technology has grown from its beginnings at the turn of the twentieth century, organizations have been formed to carry out the business of the profession. Primary responsibilities include testing, certification, representation, and education. Chapter 14 explains the role of the **American Registry of Radiologic Technologists (ARRT)** in testing and certification. This chapter highlights some of the associations to which many technologists belong.

THE AMERICAN SOCIETY OF RADIOLOGIC TECHNOLOGISTS: AN ASSOCIATION FOR ALL RADIOLOGIC SCIENCE PROFESSIONALS

The American Society of Radiologic Technologists (ASRT; www.asrt.org) was founded in 1920 by a small, dedicated group of technologists who felt the need to meet and share their knowledge with each other. It has grown from a charter membership of 46 technologists to more than 150,000 members. The ASRT is the only nationally recognized professional society that represents all radiologic technologists in the United States today.

The organization, purposes, and functions of the ASRT are directed through the bylaws of the society. The mission of the ASRT "is to advance and elevate the medical imaging and radiation therapy profession and to enhance the quality and safety of patient care."

To accomplish these aims, a well-defined organization must be in place. The House of Delegates is the governing and legislative body of the society; the board of directors must carry out the policies and procedures that are established by the house. The members of the board of directors, the president, the vice president, the president-elect, the secretary-treasurer, and the immediate past president are elected by the membership at large. All members of the board of directors must be actively employed in the field of radiologic technology.

The ASRT supports an executive office staff that carries out the wishes of the board as it serves the members. The ASRT has the following staff: executive director, vice president of communications, director of continuing education, director of customer service (who handles thousands of contacts per month), vice president of education and research, executive vice president of operations, chief financial officer, director of government relations, director of information services, director of marketing, director of public relations, executive vice president of professional development, and director of shipping and receiving.

The Board of Directors holds formal meetings throughout the year, including a mandatory meeting during the annual House of Delegates meeting to conduct the business of the ASRT. A great deal of work is also carried on by the board electronically. Serving on this board is truly a commitment of time and energy.

One of the primary reasons that the ASRT was organized was to present education and educational opportunities to the radiologic technologists of the United States, which is still a primary purpose, and the involvement is on many different levels of education.

The ASRT has been instrumental in formulating accreditation standards for the various modalities within radiologic technology. These documents are the sources for the organization and correct operation of the educational programs in the various disciplines. The ASRT has played a key role as a partner in the approval process for accreditation documents that affect educational programs in the following areas: radiography, radiation therapy, nuclear medicine, and sonography. Such documents are revised every 5 years, and the ASRT always contributes to their revision.

All educational programs in the field of radiologic technology rely heavily on the curriculum guides that the ASRT has developed for the various disciplines. These guides are written with a behavioral objective format and assist the program directors of the various programs in knowing what should be taught within the curriculum of their programs.

The ASRT provides continuing education (CE) opportunities in conjunction with the annual conference of the Radiological Society of North America (RSNA). Programs may be viewed at www.rsna.org.

Another valuable source of education for technologists is the ASRT scientific journal, *Radiologic Technology*, which is published six times each year. This journal provides radiologic technologists with the latest developments within the profession, including peer-reviewed research providing CE credit. A bimonthly newsmagazine titled the *ASRT Scanner* is also published.

The ASRT has always been committed to CE, as well as to basic education for all radiologic technologists. A reconfirmation of this commitment was the establishment of the ASRT Educational Foundation in 1984. The foundation is a separate corporation that has responsibility for all educational activities of the ASRT; it has a separate budget and depends on grants and gifts. In addition to radiologic science professionals and affiliate societies, many companies that conduct radiology-related business and that are interested in the education of radiologic technologists have contributed to the foundation. The foundation awards research grants and scholarships and sponsors self-study materials that technologists can use within their own employment setting or home to further their education. These resources include a supply of videos on various subjects, self-study booklets, and online educational opportunities.

More evidence of the commitment of the ASRT to education for radiologic technologists in the United States is the nomination of radiologic technologist trustees to the ARRT, of committee members to the Joint Review Committee on Education in Radiologic Technology (JRCERT), of committee members to the Joint Review Committee on Education in Nuclear Medicine Technology (JRCENMT), and of one committee member to the Joint Review Committee on Education in Diagnostic Medical Sonography (JRCEDMS). All of the ASRT nominees to these boards of directors represent radiologic technology.

The ASRT has been involved for many years with helping the radiologic technologist attain professional status; however, more than recognition is needed to be considered a professional. Important documents have been developed that define the fundamental role of the radiologic technologist. These documents are identified as the Practice Standards for Medical Imaging and Radiation Therapy. These standards are of extreme importance to the profession of radiologic technology and are especially pertinent to you as you define your role within the profession.

Inasmuch as being recognized as professionals by government and other agencies is both desirable and necessary for all disciplines of radiologic technology, the American College of Radiology (ACR) supports this position and recognizes the radiologic technologist as a professional member of the health care team This statement was adopted by the ACR in support of recognizing the professional status of radiologic technologists:

> *The radiologic technologist is qualified by education and the achievement of technical skills to provide patient care in diagnostic or therapeutic radiologic modalities under the direction of radiologists. In the performance of their duties, the application of proper radiologic techniques and radiation protection measures involves both initiative and independent professional judgment by the radiologic technologist (ACR, 1980).*

PRACTICE STANDARDS FOR MEDICAL IMAGING AND RADIATION THERAPY

Practice standards have been published for each of the following specialties:
Radiography
Radiation therapy
Nuclear medicine
Sonography
Magnetic resonance imaging
Mammography
Computed tomography
Cardiac interventional and vascular interventional technology
Bone densitometry
Radiologist assistant
Quality management

If professional status is to be maintained, the radiologic technologist has to do more than just be recognized as a professional; he or she must also perform in a professional manner. The measure of a professional is a very complex matter; it is the result of a combination of how we see ourselves and how our patients, our peers, and other health professionals see us. The ASRT has conducted thorough research in this area to help radiologic technologists clarify just what a professional radiologic technologist does and what constitutes professional behavior. Professionalism is a very dynamic process that must be continually practiced. Technologists must continually assess their own performance as professionals and hold themselves accountable to the patients and their peers.

SOCIOECONOMICS

The ASRT is constantly gathering data relative to staffing and compensation of radiologic technologists within the United States. The results of this data are published periodically to which members refer when negotiating for new positions or upgrading their present positions. The best source for this information is the ASRT's website at www.asrt.org.

LEGISLATION

Legislation that mandates the licensing of radiologic technologists by the states where they work has been a goal of the ASRT for decades. The members believe that the public must be protected from unnecessary exposure to radiation that is administered by people who are not adequately educated in the operation of radiation-emitting equipment. The only way to accomplish this task is to require that operators of radiation-emitting equipment be tested to ensure that they have a fundamental knowledge of radiation, its uses, and its effects.

STATE AND LOCAL AFFILIATES

Radiologic science professionals can maintain their professional involvement locally through state societies. Each state society is considered an affiliate of the ASRT and conducts its business according to ASRT standards. Most state societies conduct an annual educational conference, and many sponsor more than one such session each year.

Mandatory CE in many states has prompted the need for additional educational activities throughout the year. These sessions are generally conducted locally through districts within each state society. In addition, the members of these districts elect officials to conduct the business of the district society (e.g., publicity, fundraising, political action). Thus the goals and values of the ASRT are shared and propagated from the national to the local level.

As mentioned, the ASRT maintains an active liaison with the RSNA and the American Society for Therapeutic Radiology and Oncology (ASTRO) through joint educational and political efforts. Active communication is also maintained with the ACR, **AHRA: The Association for Medical Imaging Management**, the **Association of Collegiate Educators in Radiologic Technology (ACERT)**, and the **Association of Educators in Imaging and Radiologic Sciences (AEIRS)** to promote the common goal of safe radiology. The ASRT also has active membership in the International Society of Radiographers and Radiologic Technicians (ISRRT).

The ASRT is a multifaceted organization of, by, and for radiologic science professionals. Every radiologic technologist—as a professional—must join the organization that represents him or her and therefore contribute to the advancement of the profession. Browse the many pages of www.asrt.org to see how your professional association functions and what it offers to you.

EDUCATORS

A specialty in radiologic technology is education. Being an educator in the field today means keeping up with the latest developments in rapidly changing technology, as well as educational theory and methodology. Educational theory is one of the fastest growing specialties within radiologic technology and represents a dynamic career choice for persons who are interested in teaching the next generation of radiologic technologists.

Both the ACERT (www.acert.org) and the AEIRS (www.aeirs.org) provide forums for educators to share ideas, strategies, and solutions in their quest for excellence in radiologic science education. Although these entities are separate and distinct organizations, their primary goals are quite similar. These organizations represent several hundred program directors, clinical coordinators, and clinical instructors of radiologic technology education, and they are incorporated and governed by bylaws. The officers include a president, a president-elect, a secretary, and a treasurer.

Members may become involved by serving on one of the many committees, running for office, or presenting a paper or project at the annual conference.

Specializing in radiologic technology education is an important career decision. It requires individuals with strong communication skills, competency in the field itself, and a desire to work hard; it is also highly rewarding both professionally and personally.

RADIOLOGY MANAGERS AND SUPERVISORS

As the delivery of radiology services has become more detailed and involved, the role of the radiology administrator has also expanded. To meet their needs as radiology managers, seven administrators founded the AHRA (www.ahraonline.org) in 1973. Now a nationally recognized organization with several thousand members, the AHRA addresses the issues and concerns of this very important subspecialty of radiology.

The stated goals of the AHRA include the education and training of radiology administrators, the maintenance of high ethical standards, and communication among members. The primary focus of these goals is on the skills needed for leading people and for dealing with the changing health care environment.

The AHRA sponsors national, regional, and local meetings, and it awards continuing education units (CEUs). Written communication takes place through several publications. An annual directory provides members with names, addresses, and telephone numbers to facilitate the exchange of information among colleagues. A journal, *Radiology Management*, is published quarterly; it covers topics that are pertinent to radiology administration, such as management skills, equipment purchasing, and fiscal matters.

Also available to members are The Online Institute, providing free CE credits and an online discussion group.

Surveys are conducted by the AHRA, and the data are made available to members. Topics of such surveys have been salaries, productivity, equipment, and position descriptions, among others. By combining the knowledge of many, members have at their disposal publications that would be difficult to produce individually. The AHRA provides, for a fee, several manuals containing invaluable information and guidance to the radiology administrator.

Membership in the AHRA is open to individuals who practice radiology administration at the level of executive or department head. Other membership categories cover those who wish to contribute to the goals of the organization but who are not eligible to be active members.

It is never too early to begin considering supervision as a career in radiologic technology. Just as in patient care, people of high quality and expertise will always be necessary for leadership positions within radiology departments.

OTHER TECHNOLOGIST ORGANIZATIONS

Each specialty within radiologic technology has its own topics, concerns, and issues; therefore each has formed its own professional association. An in-depth look at each is not possible here. However, each area has as its primary goal the welfare of its patients, its members, and the profession itself.

Technologists who specialize in any aspect of radiologic technology would be wise to maintain membership in the ASRT and in whichever organizations pertain to their chosen specialty. The following professional societies currently serve more than a quarter million radiologic technologists in the United States:

AHRA: The Association for Medical Imaging Management
American Association of Medical Dosimetrists (AAMD)
American Society of Radiologic Technologists (ASRT)
Association of Collegiate Educators in Radiologic Technology (ACERT)

Association of Educators in Imaging and Radiologic Sciences (AEIRS)

Magnetic Resonance Managers Society (MRMS)

Radiology Business Management Association (RBMA)

Society for Magnetic Resonance Technologists (SMRT)

Society for Radiation Oncology Administrators (SROA)

Society of Computed Body Tomography and Magnetic Resonance (SCBTMR)

Society of Diagnostic Medical Sonographers (SDMS)

Society of Nuclear Medicine and Molecular Imaging (SNMMI)

As the field continues to grow, radiologic technologists will band together to form new associations. This networking strengthens the entire profession; it adds to the ranks of dedicated professionals who are willing to put forth the time and effort to learn, to grow, and to promote their respective specialties.

RADIOLOGIST AND PHYSICIST ORGANIZATIONS

To satisfy the needs and demands of radiologists and physicists in diagnostic imaging and therapy, several organizations have been formed over the past 100 years:

American Academy of Health Physics (AAHP)

American Academy of Oral and Maxillofacial Radiology (AAOMR)

American Association of University Radiologists (AUR)

American Association of Physicists in Medicine (AAPM)

American Association of Women Radiologists (AAWR)

American College of Medical Physics (ACMP)

American College of Nuclear Physicians (ACNP)

American College of Radiology (ACR)

American Institute of Ultrasound in Medicine (AUIM)

American Nuclear Society (ANS)

American Osteopathic College of Radiology (AOCR)

American Radium Society (ARS)

American Roentgen Ray Society (ARRS)

American Society for Therapeutic Radiology and Oncology (ASTRO)

American Society of Emergency Radiology (ASER)

American Society of Head and Neck Radiology (ASHNR)

American Society of Neuroradiology (ASNR)

Health Physics Society (HPS)

Radiation Research Society (RADRES)

Radiological Society of North America (RSNA)

Society of Breast Imaging (SBI)

Society for Pediatric Radiology (SPR)

Society of Cardiovascular and Interventional Radiology (SCVIR)

Society of Chairmen of Academic Radiation Oncology Programs (SCAROP)

Society of Chairmen of Academic Radiology Departments (SCARD)

Society of Abdominal Radiology (SAR)

Society of Nuclear Medicine (SNM)

Society of Radiologists in Ultrasound (SRU)

Society of Thoracic Radiology (STR)

In addition, the Association for Radiologic & Imaging Nursing serves nurses who work in imaging services.

CONCLUSION

Never before have so many different associations been formed within the profession; never before have true professionals been this willing to work together. As a student radiologic technologist, it is not too early to become involved at the local and state level and to join your national organization. Radiologic technology is not weaker because of specialization in imaging and therapeutic modalities, education, and administration; rather, it is stronger through diversity because each group represents a pillar of strength that supports all for which we stand.

QUESTIONS FOR DISCUSSION AND CRITICAL THINKING

1. Discuss the importance of belonging to a professional association.
2. Discuss the various aspects of the profession touched by the ASRT.
3. Explain how ACERT and AEIRS serve your instructors.
4. Explain how the AHRA serves radiology managers.

BIBLIOGRAPHY

AHRA: The Association for Medical Imaging Management. Available at http://www.ahra.org.

American Society of Radiologic Technologists. *Practice standards for medical imaging and radiation therapy.* Albuquerque. NM: Author; 2017.

Association of Collegiate Association of Collegiate Educators in Radiologic Technology. Available at http://www.acert.org.

Association of Educators Association of Educators in Imaging and Radiologic Sciences. Available at http://www.aeirs.org.

16

Clinical Specialization and Career Advancement

OBJECTIVES

On completion of this chapter, you should be able to:

- Discuss the history of the areas of specialization in radiologic technology.
- Describe the practice standards and scope of practice of the specialized areas.
- Compare upward mobility career routes for radiologic technologists.
- Determine the requirements for radiology administrators.
- Determine the requirements for radiologic technology educators.

OUTLINE

Radiologic Technology
Radiography
Computed Tomography
Magnetic Resonance Imaging
Interventional Radiography
Mammography
Bone Densitometry
Diagnostic Medical Sonography
Nuclear Medicine
Forensic Imaging Technologist

Radiation Therapy
Radiologist Assistant
Quality Assurance Technologist
Imaging Informatics: PACS Administrator
Commercial Representative
Radiology Administrator
Administrative Radiology
Radiologic Technologist Educator
Conclusion

KEY TERMS

accreditation
bone densitometry
career mobility
commercial representatives
computed tomography
CT technologist
diagnostic medical sonographer
forensic imaging
formative evaluations
imaging informatics
interventional radiology
magnetic resonance imaging

mammography
MRI technologist
nuclear medicine
nuclear medicine technologist
PACS administrator
practice standards
quality assurance technologist
quality management technologist
radiation therapist
radiation therapy
radiographers
radiologic technologist

radiologic technology
radiologic technologist educator
radiologist
radiologist assistant
radiology administrator
scope of practice
sonography
summative evaluations
surgical radiography
trauma radiography

RADIOLOGIC TECHNOLOGY

Radiologic technology is the health care field that includes diagnostic imaging modalities and radiation therapy. Whether you are already enrolled in an educational program in this field or are contemplating such a career, it is important to understand the depth and breadth of this profession.

The term "radiologic technology" may be thought of as an umbrella term that encompasses all of the specialties within this field. A radiologic technologist is a person who has been educated in and practices in one or more of these fields. To state you are is a radiologic technologist indicates you are part of this professions but does not specify the area of specialization and certification. Figure 16.1 graphically illustrates these many specialties and their specific titles.

Diagnostic radiology has progressed significantly since its beginning in 1895. It began as a means of determining a patient's illness by recording radiographic images on a photographic plate or film, identifying fractures, and examining internal organs for tumors or other physiologic disturbances. Today, however, diagnostic radiology encompasses much more than the simple procedures begun at the end of the nineteenth century.

The role of the radiologic technologist has increased in complexity and responsibility since its rather simple early beginnings. In addition to developments within diagnostic radiography, specialized areas have evolved for the diagnosis and treatment of disease. These areas, which provide many opportunities for radiologic technologists, include cardiovascular or interventional procedures, mammography, computed tomography (CT), bone densitometry, magnetic resonance imaging (MRI), nuclear medicine, diagnostic medical sonography, and radiation therapy.

Career mobility is based primarily on the formal educational background and experience of an individual. The direction of advancement and higher education needs are determined by the individual.

Student radiologic technologists interested in career mobility must examine their career priorities, assess their individual capabilities and interests, and then begin investigating pathways for success. The need for additional education depends on an individual's area of interest. Student radiologic technologists mapping their career progression must consider the time and financial investment coupled with opportunities higher education will offer them.

Many higher education programs are available for career advancement of radiologic technologists. However, in choosing a career path, an individual must determine goals and explore opportunities. In addition to the multitude of postgraduate educational opportunities are several nontraditional educational programs available to radiologic technologists. Colleges and universities offer off-campus courses as well as online courses.

Referring again to Figure 16.1, each of the specialties within radiologic technology is listed. Each has its own educational, clinical, and credentialing requirements. In addition, each has its own practice standards and scope of practice. It is important to understand these standards when considering specializing and working in these areas.

The practice standards for each area are considered guidelines for the safe practice in that field. They provide descriptions of practice criteria, education levels, and the quality of patient care expected. They are essentially job descriptions written by the profession itself.

Contained within the practice standards is the scope of practice for each specialty. The scope of practice clearly sets the boundaries of what can be done when working in that area. It is determined by the profession but can be modified by statute. It is extremely important to always be cognizant of the scope of practice and to be aware of any changes or legal modifications to it.

The American Society of Radiologic Technologists (ASRT) regularly reviews the practice standards and scopes of practice and publishes appropriate updates or modifications. Such updates may be due to the expansion of professional practice or the introduction of new technology. They may be found at www.asrt.org; search for "practice standards."

RADIOGRAPHY

Medical radiography is the largest of the radiologic technology specialties. It is where most technologists begin their career. It is a specialty that provides nearly unlimited opportunities to serve patients using x-ray technology to help provide a diagnosis and to speed the patient on to appropriate treatment.

Professionals who perform medical radiography are called radiographers. Just as a photographer is one who creates images using light, a radiographer is one who creates images using radiation. Radiographers graduate from programs ranging in length from 2 to 4 years, resulting in either associate degrees or baccalaureate degrees. Radiographers study an in-depth radiography curriculum with intensive studies and clinical experiences. Radiography is a very complex field requiring the mastering of an incalculable range of skills and knowledge. It is one of the most demanding of the health care professions. Success requires a full-time commitment to studies, culminating in graduation and passing the radiography certification examination given by the American Registry of Radiologic Technologists

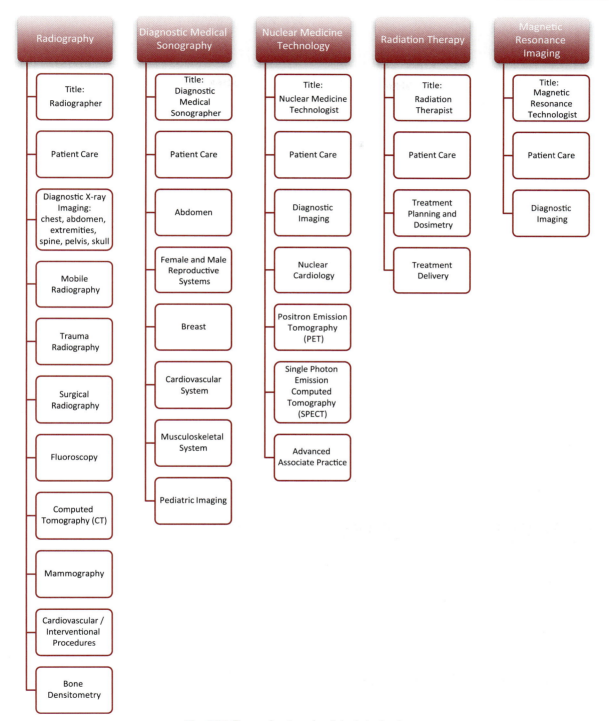

Fig. 16.1 The profession of radiologic technology.

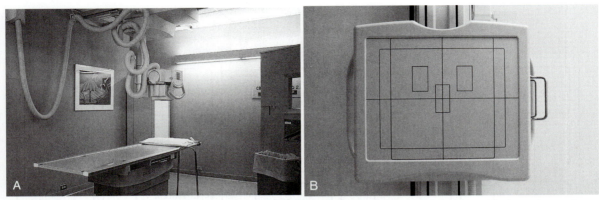

Fig. 16.2 A, A typical radiographic room. (From Long B, Rollins K, Smith B: *Merrill's atlas of radiographic positioning and procedures*, ed 14, St. Louis, 2020, Elsevier.) **B,** A wall Bucky for performing upright radiography, especially chest imaging. (From Johnston JJ, Fauber TL: *Essentials of radiographic physics and imaging*, ed 2, St. Louis, 2016, Elsevier.)

(ARRT). It is a demanding path to follow but one that offers immense personal and professional satisfaction as a career.

Radiography is performed in many different areas. Most examinations take place in a radiology department using an x-ray tube, x-ray table, and wall Bucky (Fig. 16.2). The images are captured by digital image receptors, reconstructed by computer algorithms, and displayed on a monitor (Fig. 16.3). Real-time imaging of the gastrointestinal system and other body systems is performed using a fluoroscopic unit (Fig. 16.4). The radiographer must be proficient in both radiography and fluoroscopy as well as the patient care involved.

Although the equipment and process of x-ray imaging is fascinating, the focus of the radiographer is always the patient. Patients present in many different forms with various pathologies or injuries. The radiographer specializes in caring for patients who are "routine," pediatric, obese, and geriatric (Fig. 16.5). They may be inpatients who are trying to get an accurate diagnosis or follow-up to a procedure. They may be present for an outpatient examination. The worst-case scenario is when they are there because of an accident or acute medical emergency and are part of trauma protocol. In every case, the radiographer must provide accurate images and provide the best care and service possible under the circumstances. This is what the specialty of radiography requires.

It is incumbent upon the radiographer to become so proficient at the art and science of radiography that examinations can be performed with total focus on the patient's needs and condition. The successful radiographer will eventually develop "x-ray vision," that is, the ability to visualize

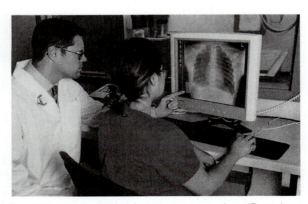

Fig. 16.3 Viewing digital images on a monitor. (From Lampignano J, Kendrick L: *Bontrager's textbook of radiographic positioning and related anatomy*, ed 9, St. Louis, 2018, Elsevier.)

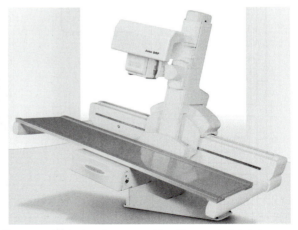

Fig. 16.4 A fluoroscopy room with a flat panel digital detector. (Courtesy of Philips Healthcare. All rights reserved.)

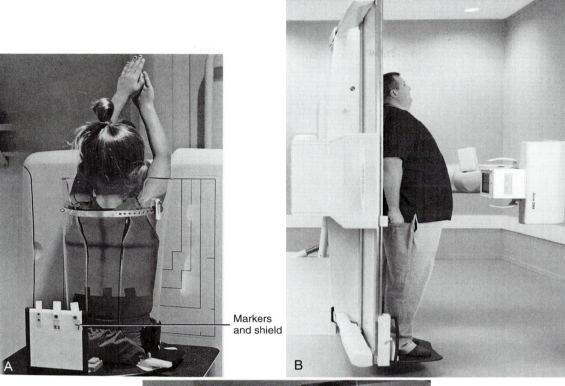

Markers
and shield

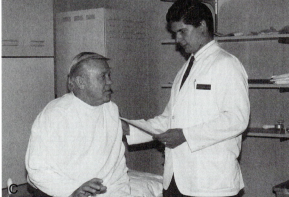

Fig. 16.5 A, Pediatric chest imaging with patient positioned in a Pigg-O-Stat. (From Lampignano J, Kendrick L: *Bontrager's textbook of radiographic positioning and related anatomy*, ed 9, St. Louis, 2018, Elsevier.) **B,** Radiography of an obese patient. (From Long B, Rollins K, Smith B: *Merrill's atlas of radiographic positioning and procedures,* ed 14, St. Louis, 2020, Elsevier.) **C,** Carefully explaining an examination to a geriatric patient. (From Long B, Rollins K, Smith B: *Merrill's atlas of radiographic positioning and procedures*, ed 14, St. Louis, 2020, Elsevier.)

how the image will appear before even making the exposure. This talent enables highly accurate patient positioning and optimal exposure technique. It comes with time and experience.

Radiography is not confined to the radiology department. The need for x-ray imaging exists in other locations. Radiographers may spend part of their shift outside of the radiology department. For patients who are unable to be transported to the radiology department, radiographers take a mobile, or portable, x-ray machine to the patient. The patient may be in a regular hospital room, postanesthesia care unit, intensive care unit, coronary care unit, neonatal intensive care unit, or burn unit. In every case, the radiographer performing mobile radiography must be prepared to acquire accurate, diagnostic images while working within a very demanding environment.

A stressful environment that must be mastered by a radiographer is **surgical radiography**. The best surgeons do not possess x-ray vision. They depend on the radiographer operating a portable x-ray machine or a portable fluoroscope, also known as a C-arm (Fig. 16.6), to provide clear images during an operation. These operations usually involve repairing fractures, inserting new joints, or any other work requiring x-ray images to verify the accuracy of the surgical procedure. To work in an operating room, the radiographer must be in full surgical attire (Fig. 16.7) and completely understand sterile technique and sterile fields.

Perhaps the examinations requiring the most speed and accuracy involve trauma. Patients who are brought to an emergency department (ED) are normally in need of immediate care. Just as a surgeon does not have x-ray vision, the best ED physicians and nurses cannot provide care until

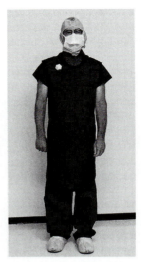

Fig. 16.7 Radiographer properly attired for work in the operating suite. (From Lampignano J, Kendrick L: *Bontrager's textbook of radiographic positioning and related anatomy*, ed 9, St. Louis, 2018, Elsevier.)

they have a diagnosis. In most cases, the diagnosis is provided by a radiologist interpreting the images acquired by a radiographer. The radiographer plays a crucial role in trauma cases. A comprehensive knowledge of radiographic positioning and all its variations is required. Often normal positioning of a part cannot take place because of injury. The radiographer must be able to vary those positions and x-ray tube angles to obtain the best image possible to use for a diagnosis. Speed is of the utmost importance; accuracy is critical. Although being a high-stress situation, **trauma radiography** is very fulfilling because of its role in caring for seriously ill or injured patients.

As can be seen here, the specialty of radiography is both fulfilling and demanding. It is far reaching in its care for patients, and it plays a major role in bringing patients back to well-being. It can be used as a stepping stone to other radiologic technology specialties, or it can be an extremely rewarding specialty as a radiographer.

COMPUTED TOMOGRAPHY

Computed tomography, which is the gathering of anatomic information from a cross-sectional plane of the body and presenting it as a three-dimensional (3D) image, was introduced in 1972 at the annual congress of the British Institute of Radiology by G.N. Hounsfield, a senior research scientist at EMI Limited in Middlesex, England. A CT image is formed by scanning a thin cross-section of the body with a narrow x-ray beam and measuring the

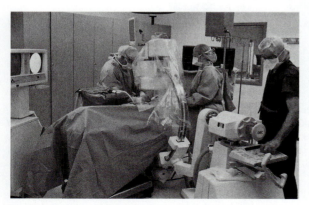

Fig. 16.6 Fluoroscopy in a surgical suite using a C-arm with careful attention to sterile fields. (From Lampignano J, Kendrick L: *Bontrager's textbook of radiographic positioning and related anatomy*, ed 9, St. Louis, 2018, Elsevier.)

transmitted radiation with a special detector. The detector does not form the image by itself. The information is numeric in form and is then processed by a computer to construct an image.

A CT radiographer, or **CT technologist**, must be able to perform CT procedures without constant supervision of technical detail. The technologist must have a thorough knowledge of anatomy, especially in cross-section. Judgments about the formation of the image may have to be made without the direct guidance of a radiologist. Equipment must be maintained and kept orderly, and any mechanical difficulties must be reported for service. The technologist must maintain visual and audible contact with the patient during the examination and observe for unusual emergency situations. Knowledge of sterile technique in administering contrast media is essential for the technologist (Fig. 16.8), and all emergency equipment must be maintained in case of a reaction to contrast media. In addition, a complete history of each patient must be recorded.

Most CT units have three functional components involved in the production of an image: the scanning unit, the computer, and the viewing unit. The scanning unit uses a very small beam. After the beam has passed through the body, it is picked up by a detector that produces an electric signal in proportion to the intensity of the x-ray beam. A profile of the body section is obtained by moving the x-ray beam over the body or by simultaneously using several

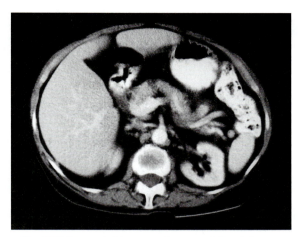

Fig. 16.9 Computed tomography scan of the abdomen.

beams. Within the CT system is a computer that forms the image from the multiple x-ray beams; this process is mathematical, and the image created is numeric. For viewing, the numeric image is converted into a video signal that is displayed on a monitor; the video signal is represented by varying shades of gray. Very dense structures are demonstrated as white areas; less dense structures are dark gray (Fig. 16.9). CT has made possible the diagnosis of disease processes of organs such as the liver and pancreas that, before this time, could not be demonstrated by normal radiographic methods. Also, because the image is digital, it may be post-processed for viewing from many angles and reconstructed into three dimensions if necessary.

Although the first scanners were designed for evaluating the brain, now any part of the body can be scanned by CT systems. In addition, contrast media can be administered to highlight any low-contrast areas.

Although some colleges offer CT education, many CT technologists are radiographers who have been cross trained in a clinical setting. They have documented their clinical experiences and have become credentialed by the ARRT. It is extremely important to acquire ARRT certification when working in CT.

Many opportunities are available for CT radiographers in hospitals and clinics. See Box 16.1 for career information.

MAGNETIC RESONANCE IMAGING

Magnetic resonance imaging was introduced in the early 1980s. Originally, MRI was called nuclear magnetic resonance (NMR). The word *nuclear* caused some confusion because of the association with radioactive materials used in nuclear medicine; therefore it was discontinued because no nuclear radiation is involved. NMR had been around for

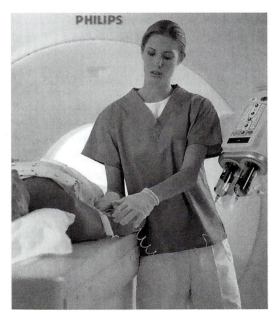

Fig. 16.8 Computed tomography technologist preparing to inject a contrast agent. (Courtesy of Philips Healthcare. All rights reserved.)

quite some time because it was used in chemistry and physics to obtain information about complex molecules and molecular motion.

The equipment used for MRI consists of large electromagnetic coils that surround a second electromagnetic coil that is capable of delivering pulses of radio waves. The patient lies inside the hollow, cylindrically arranged magnetic coils and is subjected to a magnetic field that is thousands of times more powerful than the earth's magnetic field. When the magnetic field acts on the patient's body, the nuclei of the body's atoms—particularly of the hydrogen atoms—arrange themselves parallel to each other similar to rows of tiny magnets. Normally, the spinning atoms' nuclei point randomly in different directions. When the patient is in the magnetic field, some of the spinning hydrogen nuclei line up in the same direction as the polarity of the magnetic waves. At this instant, a pulse of radio waves is emitted by the second inside electromagnetic coil; this emission causes the spinning nuclei within the tissue to change their angle of rotation because of the absorbed energy of the radiofrequency pulse. The wobbles produced by the changing angles of rotation produce signals that are analyzed to produce an image that shows varying densities of hydrogen in the body part.

Magnetic resonance imaging provides cross-sectional, 3D images and functional studies without using x-rays or radioactive materials; it produces images with the use of a strong magnetic field and radio waves. Hence, there is no risk sometimes associated with ionizing radiation.

An **MRI technologist** must be able to perform MRI procedures without constant supervision of technical detail. As in other imaging modalities, they must have a thorough knowledge of anatomy, especially in cross-section. Judgments about the MRI pulsing sequence, gradient magnetic fields, and anatomic slice orientation must be made.

Knowledge about the characteristics of magnetic fields, electromagnets, and atomic structure is important in MRI. A computer is used in magnetic imaging, just as one is used in CT, and thus a basic knowledge of how a computer

constructs the image is required. Patient care responsibilities apply in MRI very much the same as in other types of diagnostic imaging. Knowledge of sterile technique in the administration of contrast media is needed, and all emergency equipment must be maintained in case of a patient reaction.

The MRI produces images of body parts that are surrounded by bone in clear, unobstructed detail; this characteristic makes it especially useful for studying the brain and spinal cord (Fig. 16.10). MRI can show the detail of nerve damage by such diseases as multiple sclerosis; it can also detect brain tumors that may be obscured by bone in other imaging procedures.

An obvious disadvantage in the MRI scanning exists. Because the body is placed in a strong magnetic field, metallic objects on the patient (e.g., jewelry), as well as in the patient (e.g., hip joint prosthesis plates, screws in bones, surgical clips), are also affected by the magnet.

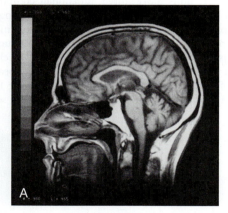

A

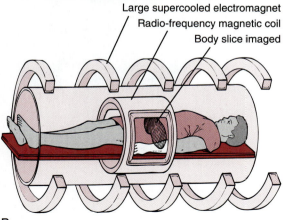

Large supercooled electromagnet
Radio-frequency magnetic coil
Body slice imaged

B

Fig. 16.10 A and **B,** Since its inception in the 1980s, magnetic resonance imaging has become a routine diagnostic modality.

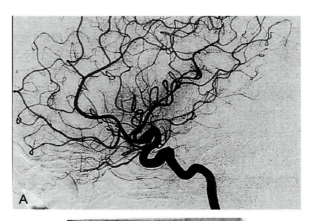

Although some colleges offer MRI education, many MR technologists are radiographers who have been cross trained in a clinical setting. They have documented their clinical experiences and have become credentialed by the ARRT. It is extremely important to acquire ARRT certification when working in MRI.

Many opportunities are available for MR technologists in hospitals and clinics. See Box 16.2 for career information.

INTERVENTIONAL RADIOGRAPHY

Special procedures radiography, as it was once called, began soon after Roentgen's discovery of x-radiation. One of the most successful early investigators was Walter Bradford Cannon, who began his work in 1896 when he was still a medical student. Cannon placed animals that had ingested radiopaque buttons and balls in front of an x-ray tube and followed the movement of the digestive tract. Eventually, he used barium sulfate suspension, which is still used today, to study the digestive system.

By 1920, investigators began to develop agents that produced contrast in specific organs. As more complicated procedures were developed, these examinations quickly became the routine daily diagnostic contrast procedures used in radiology departments.

Interventional radiology, as it is now called, has evolved to include diagnostic and treatment procedures primarily of the heart and vascular system. Angiograms provide detailed images of select areas of the circulatory system. Cardiac catheterization for diagnosis and treatment of the heart is part of this specialty as is stroke detection and treatment.

Many examinations may be included under special procedures radiography; however, studies of the circulatory system are generally considered the most common.

Angiography refers to the study of the circulatory structures by opacifying the blood vessels with a positive contrast medium (Fig. 16.11). Many different angiographic studies are performed in a radiology department; the examination

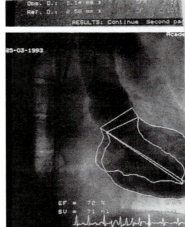

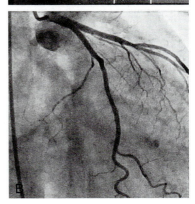

Fig. 16.11 **A,** Left lateral internal carotid arteriogram. **B,** Left coronary artery imaged during cardiac catheterization. (Courtesy of Philips Healthcare. All rights reserved.)

is identified by the particular vascular structure demonstrated and the method of injection of contrast media.

Arteriography is the study of arterial vessels, which may be broken down further into peripheral studies of the extremities and visceral studies of various organs in the chest or abdomen. Venography is the study of the venous system, cerebral angiography is the examination of the vessels in the brain; angiocardiography is the opacification of the heart and great vessels, and aortography is the study of the thoracic or abdominal aorta.

Injection of contrast media can be made directly into the vessel of interest or indirectly through another vessel through a catheter. Contrast media can be injected by hand, but most frequently, an electromechanical or compressed air device, called a pressure injector, is used.

Angiographic studies are performed to demonstrate any vascular abnormalities or pathologic conditions in the surrounding tissue and organs, such as tumors. Examinations are also performed to demonstrate organ function, as in a study of the heart valves or kidneys.

Accessory equipment other than radiographic equipment is needed for interventional radiography. Monitoring devices that record electric impulses of the heart and pressure within the heart and great vessels are often used. Anesthesia equipment might be necessary, as well as an emergency apparatus such as a crash cart that contains drugs, defibrillators, suction machines, and other resuscitation devices.

Interventional radiology procedures require not only specialized equipment (Fig. 16.12) but also a highly trained team to successfully perform the techniques required to obtain optimal diagnostic information. The interventional radiologic technologist is an important part of this team and is responsible for operating the equipment, making preparations for the procedures and assisting the physician during the examination. Extensive knowledge of the heart and

> ### BOX 16.3   Careers in Interventional Radiography
>
> For information on a career in interventional radiography, visit the American Society of Radiologic Technologists: www.asrt.org
>
> For a listing of educational programs in interventional radiography, use any comprehensive Internet search engine, such as Google (search by topic)
>
> For information on the certification exam in interventional radiography, visit the American Registry of Radiologic Technologists: www.arrt.org

circulatory system is mandatory. In addition, the technologist must be fluent in cardiac monitoring and sterile technique.

An interventional technologist performs radiographic procedures of a highly technical nature without supervision of technical detail. This position requires thorough knowledge of the highly sophisticated equipment.

Most interventional radiographers have been cross trained in a clinical setting. Schools offering education in interventional procedures radiography are usually baccalaureate degree programs. Registered radiologic technologists may apply to sit for the ARRT examination in interventional radiography.

Employment opportunities vary. Most special procedures are performed in large hospitals and medical clinics. Salaries vary by location and employer. See Box 16.3 for career information.

MAMMOGRAPHY

Breast cancer is a major condition that affects our female population, although some males are affected by it as well (Fig. 16.13). Increased chances for a cure depend on early detection.

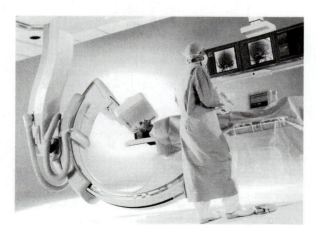

Fig. 16.12 Flat panel detector digital angiographic system, single plane. (Courtesy of Philips Healthcare. All rights reserved.)

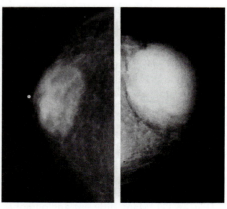

Fig. 16.13 Invasive ductal cancer in a male patient. (Modified from Ikeda DM: *Breast imaging*, St. Louis, 2005, Mosby.)

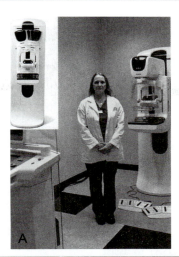

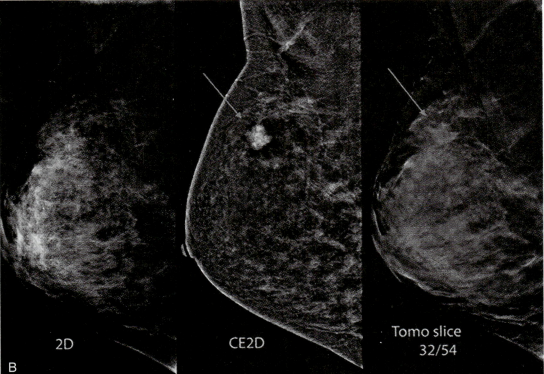

2D   CE2D   Tomo slice
                      32/54

B

Fig. 16.14 **A,** Mammographer with a three-dimensional (3D) breast tomosynthesis unit. (Courtesy of SimonMed Imaging, Scottsdale, AZ. Inset, Courtesy of Hologic, Bedford, MA.) **B,** 3D image of the breast. (Courtesy of Hologic.)

Mammography, which is the radiographic examination of the breast, is a specialized discipline because the nature of breast tissue requires unique technical procedures. A dedicated radiographic unit and equipment are required for optimal diagnostic results. Such equipment has advanced to the stage of producing 3D images for even more accurate diagnosis (Fig. 16.14).

Radiographers who specialize in mammography are called mammographers. They must have a detailed knowledge of breast anatomy. Their positioning of the breast on the dedicated mammography unit must be precise. Image acquisition is required to be highly accurate. In addition, mammographers must have a thorough knowledge of the Mammography Quality Standards Act (MQSA) to assist in keeping the mammography department properly accredited and certified.

Although some colleges offer mammography programs, most mammographers are radiographers who have been cross trained in a clinical setting. They have documented their clinical experiences and have become credentialed by the ARRT. It is extremely important to acquire ARRT certification when working in mammography.

Many opportunities are available for mammographers in hospitals and outpatient clinics. See Box 16.4 for career information.

BONE DENSITOMETRY

Bone densitometry plays an important role in detecting and treating osteoporosis. Special equipment is required for bone densitometry (Fig. 16.15). It makes use of radiation and is specially designed to measure bone mineral density.

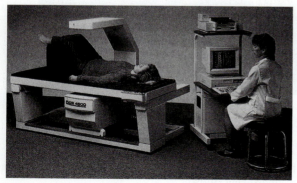

Fig. 16.15 Bone densitometry of the spine. (Courtesy of Hologic, Bedford, MA.)

Bone health, particularly of patients in whom osteoporosis is suspected, can be evaluated this way.

Extensive knowledge of the bone densitometry equipment and human anatomy, particularly bone anatomy, are required. Radiation safety and a complete understanding of image acquisition and reconstruction is vital.

Most bone densitometry technologists have been cross trained in a clinical setting by the employer and manufacturer of the equipment. They have documented their clinical experiences and have become credentialed by the ARRT. It is extremely important to acquire ARRT certification when working in bone densitometry.

Opportunities are available for bone densitometry technologists in hospitals and orthopedic clinics. See Box 16.5 for career information.

DIAGNOSTIC MEDICAL SONOGRAPHY

Diagnostic medical **sonography**, which is often called *ultrasound*, uses high-frequency sound waves to form an image. A sound beam is similar to an x-ray beam in that it is composed of waves that transfer energy from one point to another. Radiation passes through a vacuum, but sound waves can pass only through matter. Sound waves are simply vibrations that pass through a material. If no material exists, nothing is available to vibrate, and therefore sound cannot exist.

Sonography was first successfully used during World War I to detect submarines but not until after World War II did testing begin on human tissue for diagnostic purposes. In the late 1940s and early 1950s, three physicians—working independently—discovered that if ultrasound waves were sent through the body, echoes reflected from the different tissues would return and could form an image of the anatomic structures, and a permanent photograph could be made of the image.

The components necessary to produce an ultrasonic image are a transducer, an ultrasound beam, and an image display on a video monitor (Fig. 16.16). The transducer

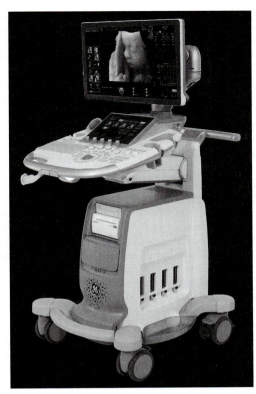

Fig. 16.16 Ultrasound unit. (Used with permission of GE Healthcare.)

serves two purposes: (1) it transmits sound in pulses or bursts (~2000–15,000/second), and (2) it senses the echoes that are returning from the previous pulse. The **diagnostic medical sonographer** positions the transducer on the patient and applies it to the area of interest to produce echoes while adjusting the monitor controls to achieve the optimal image. The electronic image is made one bit at a time from each returning echo and is displayed as a video image. The sonographer must have a thorough knowledge of anatomy and pathology to be able to interpret the images as they appear on the monitor.

X-rays are produced when electrons are accelerated to a very high speed and then decelerated or suddenly stopped. Sound waves are produced in the transducer by a vibrating crystal. When the transducer is placed in contact with the body, the vibrating crystal causes the particles in the body to vibrate; the vibrations are then passed from one layer of tissue to another. Reflections of the ultrasound pulses are created at the borders between two different body structures. With both ultrasound and radiographic images, adjacent structures to be visualized must differ in physical

characteristics, such as atomic number or thickness. One significant difference between sonography and radiography is that whereas an ultrasound pulse continually loses energy as it passes through the body, an x-ray photon loses its energy all at once.

The first sonograms were incomplete; they were not two-dimensional (2D) images. Immersing the patient in a tank of water improved the image, but the biggest improvement came with the development of compound scanning, in which the transducer is moved simultaneously in two different patterns over the area of interest. A lubricating gel is placed on the patient's skin, thereby minimizing friction and air gaps between the skin surface and the transducer and enhancing the image.

A diagnostic medical sonographer performs various ultrasound examinations for the diagnosis of tumors, the malfunction of organs, and evaluation during pregnancy (Fig. 16.17). Any soft tissue area of the body may be examined with the use of ultrasound—from abdominal organs to the evaluation of blood flow.

Several options for education in sonography are available. Educational programs in sonography may be 1½, 2, or 4 years in length, depending on the curriculum offered and the inclusion of earned credit hours for an academic degree. The course of study involves biology, sectional anatomy, patient care, physics and equipment of sonography, diagnostic procedures, imaging, and image evaluation. Clinical education also constitutes a major portion of the program. Upon graduation, a candidate may apply to take certification examinations administered by the American Registry of Diagnostic Medical Sonographers or the ARRT.

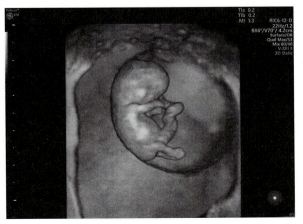

Fig. 16.17 Obstetric scan, first trimester. (Used with permission of GE Healthcare.)

A diagnostic medical sonographer is qualified to work in a hospital, clinic, or private practice. Salaries vary according to location, employer, and work experience. See Box 16.6 for career information.

NUCLEAR MEDICINE

Radioactivity, which was co-discovered by Marie Curie, Pierre Curie, and Henri Becquerel in 1898, is a phenomenon in which the nucleus of an atom contains excess energy and is considered excited or unstable; the nucleus spontaneously emits this energy in the form of radiation to reach a more stable state. The three types of rays emitted are alpha, beta, and gamma. Alpha and beta particles are small pieces of the nucleus that have been ejected. Gamma rays are identical to x-rays except that they originate from the nucleus of an unstable atom; x-rays are generated in a radiographic tube.

Radioactive elements can be naturally occurring or artificially produced in cyclotrons and nuclear reactors. All of the radioactive compounds used in **nuclear medicine**, often called *radionuclides* or *radiopharmaceuticals*, are artificially produced.

Radiopharmaceuticals are used as tracers in nuclear medicine studies. A tracer is a substance that emits radiation and that can be identified when placed in the human body. By detecting the tracer, information about the structure, function, secretion, excretion, and volume of a particular organ can be obtained.

A **nuclear medicine technologist** provides physicians with essential molecular-level information about both the structure and the function of organs and body systems. Using small amounts of radioactive materials administered to the patient by oral, intravenous, subcutaneous, direct introduction, or any combination, nuclear medicine imaging and analysis provides essential information to a broad range of medical specialties, including cardiology, oncology, psychiatry, and pediatrics. The use of nuclear medicine procedures often permits earlier identification of abnormalities, thus permitting more timely diagnosis and effective treatment. New and developing diagnostic and therapeutic procedures are revolutionizing the understanding of a host of diseases and conditions.

Nuclear medicine imaging equipment works with computers, producing images and data used to detect and analyze the biodistribution of radionuclides and radiopharmaceuticals in the body. Both 2D planar and 3D tomographic (single-photon emission computed tomography [SPECT] [Fig. 16.18] and positron emission tomography [PET]) images are acquired in nuclear medicine.

Nuclear medicine may be used for diagnostic and therapeutic studies both inside (in vivo) and outside (in vitro) the body. The nuclear medicine technologist prepares and administers radiopharmaceuticals to patients by intravenous, intramuscular, subcutaneous, and oral methods and also manages the quality control of the substances. The nuclear medicine technologist must understand and use radiation detection devices and other laboratory equipment that measure the quantity and distribution of radionuclides deposited in a patient or in a patient's specimen. In addition, in vivo and in vitro procedures must be performed safely by applying the principles of radiation protection to limit the amount of radiation exposure to the patient, the public, and other employees.

Educational programs in nuclear medicine technology may be 1, 2, or 4 years in length, depending on the curriculum offered and the inclusion of earned credit hours for an academic degree. The course of study involves biology, anatomy, patient care, nuclear physics and instrumentation, computer technology, biochemistry, radiopharmacology, radiation biology and health physics, radiation protection, immunology, radionuclide therapy, and statistics. Diagnostic procedures, imaging, and image evaluation, including extensive clinical education, also constitute a major portion of the program. Upon completion of the nuclear medicine education program, a student is eligible to apply for testing by the ARRT or the Nuclear Medicine Technology Certification Board.

Opportunities for employment are varied and include hospitals, clinics, nuclear pharmacies, research facilities, and mobile imaging services. Salaries may vary according to location, employer, work experience, and level of education. See Box 16.7 for career information.

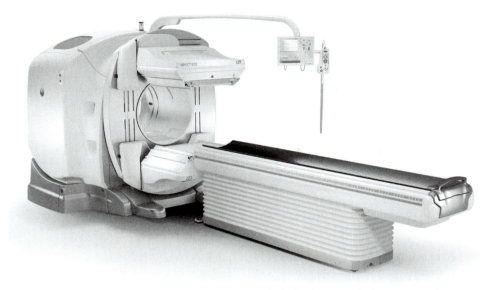

Fig. 16.18 Fusion imaging unit, computed tomography and single-photon emission computed tomography. (Used with permission of GE Healthcare.)

FORENSIC IMAGING TECHNOLOGIST

Forensics has emerged as yet another specialty for radiographers. Forensic radiology uses imaging to assist pathologists, and in some cases anthropologists, identify remains or to verify the cause of death.

The virtual autopsy, also known as virtopsy, makes use of 3D CT or MRI to image the remains. Such technology can also be used for facial reconstruction to assist with identification of a body that cannot be identified any other way due to lack of dental records or in cases of extreme malformation or decomposition. **Forensic imaging** also plays a major role in cases of child abuse.

Moving into the role of a forensic imaging technologist requires extensive experience as a radiographer with CT or MRI as additional specialties. Offering to work as a forensic assistant at a hospital department of pathology or morgue is a gateway into this field. Knowledge of the law as it pertains to forensics is mandatory.

The American Academy of Forensic Sciences website (www.aafs.org), in addition to containing extensive information on the field, also provides a list of colleges and universities offering bachelor's and master's degrees in various aspect of forensics.

RADIATION THERAPY

Radiation therapy, which may also be called *radiation oncology*, began approximately 1 year after x-rays were discovered in 1895. A medical student, Emil H. Grubbe, together with a physician friend, treated an advanced case of breast cancer with x-rays in 1896. Grubbe continued his research for many years but eventually contracted skin cancer and lost his left hand. Neither radiation nor its potential dangers were yet fully understood. Rather, radiation was thought to be a cure-all. After discovering that radiation produced epilation (loss of hair), the suggestion was made that shaving would no longer be necessary. Radiation was also used to cure blindness, epilepsy, acne, and warts, as well as various bacterial and viral infections. Almost every form of malignant and benign disease was treated. Because so little was known about the effects of radiation, the results were disappointing. The damaging effects of radiation were realized as the number of injuries was brought to public attention. Some people even demanded that the use of radiation be abandoned altogether, but techniques and equipment improved, with an increasing number of good results.

In 1904, Bergonie and Tribondeau announced their landmark findings about tissue response to radiation. They discovered that, at certain times, living cells are more sensitive to the effects of radiation. Cells that are immature, nonspecialized, and rapidly dividing are very radiosensitive. This finding was key to treating cancer with radiation.

Unlike the other specializations in radiology, radiation therapy is not used to diagnose disease. Therapy involves treating a patient who is already known to have a disease. Radiation therapy is practiced by exposing a diseased area to various types of radiation while also trying to protect the unaffected parts of the patient's body from radiation exposure. Most of the diseases treated with radiation today are cancerous. In the past, nonmalignant diseases were successfully treated with radiation, but today other forms of therapy are preferable for most noncancerous conditions.

A **radiation therapist** applies ionizing radiation to the patient in accordance with the prescription and instructions of the radiation oncologist, a physician specializing in the treatment of cancer with radiation (Fig. 16.19). Accurate technical details of treatment administered must be recorded at the time of treatment. The patient must be properly positioned, and the area of interest must be correctly marked. In addition, the radiation therapist assists in the calibration of equipment and must be able to detect malfunctions and maintain control if a radiation accident occurs. The radiation therapist may be required to prepare molds and casts of various body parts, and he or she must understand the use of wedge and compensating filters for treatment. An understanding of minor surgical procedures and aseptic technique may also be required.

Just as important, radiation therapists must render care and comfort to the patient. Unlike diagnostic radiography, in which the radiographer has brief contact with patients, patients undergoing radiation therapy are seen on a regular basis. Because of the traumatic emotional aspects that may be associated with a patient who is undergoing treatment for a malignancy, the radiation therapist must be empathetic to patients' needs and refer them, when necessary, to social services.

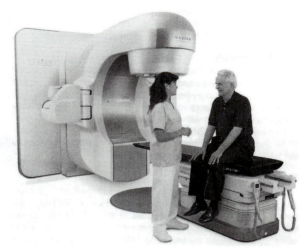

Fig. 16.19 Linear accelerator used in radiation therapy. (Image courtesy of Varian Medical Systems, Inc. All rights reserved.)

Educational programs in radiation therapy technology may be 1, 2, or 4 years in length depending on the curriculum offered and the inclusion of earned credit hours for an academic degree. The course of study involves biology, radiation oncology, pathology, radiation biology, physics and equipment of radiation therapy, intensity modulated radiation therapy, dosimetry, computer technology, and quality assurance. At the successful completion of the educational program, a student is eligible to apply to take the certification examination offered by the ARRT. On successful completion of the examination, a certified radiation therapist is qualified to work in any major cancer treatment center or in large hospitals that have both diagnostic equipment and high-energy radiation therapy units. Individual state licensure may also be required. See Box 16.8 for career information.

BOX 16.8   Careers in Radiation Therapy

For information on a career as a radiation therapist, visit the American Society of Radiologic Technologists: www.asrt.org

For a listing of accredited educational programs in radiation therapy, visit The Joint Review Committee on Education in Radiologic Technology: www.jrcert.org

For information on the certification exam in radiation therapy, visit the American Registry of Radiologic Technologists: www.arrt.org

---

BOX 16.9   Careers in Medical Dosimetry

For information on a career in medical dosimetry, visit:
   American Society of Radiologic Technologists: www.asrt.org
   American Association of Medical Dosimetrists: www.medicaldosimetry.org
For a listing of accredited educational programs in medical dosimetry, visit:
   American Association of Medical Dosimetrists: www.medicaldosimetry.org
For information on the certification exam in medical dosimetry, visit:
   Medical Dosimetrist Certification Board: www.mdcb.org

BOX 16.10   Radiologist Assistant Careers

For information on a career as a radiologist assistant, visit:
   American Society of Radiologic Technologists: www.asrt.org
   American College of Radiology: www.acr.org
For a listing of accredited educational programs in radiologist assistant, visit:
   American Society of Radiologic Technologists: www.asrt.org
For information on the certification exam in radiologist assistant, visit:
   American Registry of Radiologic Technologists: www.arrt.org

---

A certified radiation therapist may also wish to pursue additional education in medical dosimetry. A dosimetrist plans patient treatments and analyzes the radiation distribution and dose for accuracy and safety. Additional training can be up to 2 years of academics and 1 year of supervised work experience under a certified medical dosimetrist or certified medical physicist before examination by the Medical Dosimetrist Certification Board (MDCB). See Box 16.9 for career information.

Opportunities for employment are available throughout the country. Positions are generally found in larger clinics or medical centers. Salaries vary according to location, employer, education, and work experience.

RADIOLOGIST ASSISTANT

In the 1990s, a shortage of practicing radiologists was growing and by the early part of the twenty-first century, the shortage became a reality. In the summer of 2002, the American College of Radiology (ACR) decided to move forward in developing, along with the ASRT and the ARRT, the **radiologist assistant** (RA) concept as a physician-extender specifically for radiologists. The ASRT developed a standardized curriculum to include patient assessment, management and education, pharmacology, radiation safety, radiobiology, health physics, pathophysiology, and clinical preceptorship.

The RA is an advanced-level radiologic technologist who works under the supervision of a radiologist to assist in the diagnostic imaging clinical environment. The RA is an ARRT-certified radiographer who has successfully completed an advanced academic program. The programs, although limited in number, offer a nationally recognized RA curriculum and a radiologist-directed clinical preceptorship.

The focus of the RA is to perform select radiology procedures, including (but not limited to) fluoroscopy and patient assessment and management, as well as patient education. RAs participate in the systematic analysis of the quality of patient care delivered within the radiology environment. RAs also make initial observations of diagnostic images, with official interpretations and written reports being supervised by the radiologist (as defined by the ACR standards for communication in diagnostic radiology).

Education of radiologist assistants is based at the baccalaureate and postbaccalaureate levels.

See Box 16.10 for career information.

QUALITY ASSURANCE TECHNOLOGIST

The health care industry stresses accountability and commitment to the patient-centered practice. Awareness of this responsibility has caused many hospitals to voluntarily submit to **accreditation**, which is a process that a health care institution, provider, or program undergoes to demonstrate compliance with the standards developed by an official agency known as The Joint Commission (TJC). Such accreditation demands every department within the hospital meet specific standards.

The imaging department is required to meet very stringent standards regarding the delivery of ionizing radiation to the patient. These standards require that the radiology department have a quality assurance program. Quality assurance refers to the total delivery of imaging services and will include quality control, which refers to the quality and safety of the imaging equipment itself. The **quality assurance technologist** has the responsibility to guarantee that equipment meets the standards set not only by TJC, but also by federal, state, and local standards.

The quality assurance technologist, also called the **quality management technologist**, is often a radiologic technologist with a baccalaureate degree or a master's degree with specialization in physics, radiation health physics, medical physics, or occupational safety. Such degree requirements vary by employer. Also vital to this role is extensive experience as a radiographer.

IMAGING INFORMATICS: PACS ADMINISTRATOR

Informatics may be thought of as information gathering and engineering. It documents the interactions among people, technologies, systems, and organizations. Consequently, it is far reaching, especially in a field such as radiology, in which patient information, imaging, diagnoses, reports, and billing are all processed digitally.

The picture archiving and communication system (PACS) is the heart of **imaging informatics**. It blends clinical information, including diagnostic images, with documentation such as patient history, electronic medical record, diagnosis, and physician reports.

The **PACS administrator** must have a thorough understanding of imaging, human anatomy and physiology, pathology, and computer technology including networking. The field requires full comprehension of the interface between the hospital information system (HIS) and the radiology information system (RIS). This technologist must also understand DICOM (digital imaging and communications in medicine), which allows the various imaging modalities to communicate, as well as HL7 (health level seven), which provides for the integration of electronic health data. Imaging informatics provides for the efficient management of imaging services, proper patient care, and accurate billing for services.

Working in imaging informatics includes passing the Certified Imaging Informatics Professional (CIIP) examination administered by the American Board of Imaging Informatics (ABII). The ABII was founded by the Society for Imaging Informatics in Medicine (SIIM) and the ARRT.

See Box 16.11 for career information.

BOX 16.11   Careers in Imaging Informatics

For information on a career in imaging informatics, visit the Society for Imaging Informatics in Medicine: www.siim.org

For information on the certification exam in imaging informatics, visit the American Board of Imaging Informatics: www.abii.org

---

COMMERCIAL REPRESENTATIVE

Commercial representatives of various equipment companies are frequent visitors to radiology departments. The category of commercial representative could probably be best divided into two groups: applications specialists and sales representatives. A technical background is important for applications specialists because they deal with the professional staff regarding new equipment and the applications of that equipment to a particular area of radiology and imaging sciences. Their background allows them to discuss in a knowledgeable fashion the technical use of the equipment in the production of a quality image.

Sales representatives possess a baccalaureate degree and a business background. Their interactions are primarily with the radiology administrator, radiologist, and other hospital administrators. Commercial representatives should possess a high degree of maturity and confidence; in addition, they should also be able to communicate well and be committed to the products that they are selling or representing.

Many companies provide a training program for individuals who are coming into the commercial field without a previous sales or applications background; this type of program provides support during a very crucial transition period. Commercial representatives may be required to travel a great deal with their job so as to cover extensive territories. In addition, they may be asked to relocate and be reassigned to an area where their expertise is needed. Many of the commercial representatives are salaried employees, but others are commissioned employees.

RADIOLOGY ADMINISTRATOR

In the past, the department of radiology was a small, contained unit within the hospital that was easily managed by a chief radiologic technologist whose expertise was primarily in the technical area. However, the department of radiology has become a large department that employs numerous professional and nonprofessional staff members and requires an expanded budget. In addition, the regulations specified by federal and state authorities of radiation control must be met, and detailed planning for future departmental expansion is always on the drawing board. Because the traditional chief radiologic technologist cannot have expertise in all of these areas, the demand has grown for individuals with business and management backgrounds to administer the department of radiology.

The ideal **radiology administrator** has a combined technical and management background, thereby possessing both radiologic expertise and management training or experience. This position is involved in purchasing, personnel management, union negotiations, budget preparation, regulatory specifications, decision making, and planning.

Individuals pursuing radiology and imaging sciences administration can pursue higher education programs in health care administration; many colleges offer degree programs in this area. Courses in health care administration might include principles of management, statistics, industrial relations or personnel management, financial accounting, health care administration, health planning, and legal aspects of health services administration. Some institutions require a clinical management practicum. Such courses lead to a baccalaureate degree in health care management. A baccalaureate degree is the minimal requirement in radiologic and imaging sciences administration. The majority of individuals in administration hold graduate or postgraduate degrees.

Although certifications have traditionally been available in the various radiologic technology specialties, a void existed in managerial certification. In other radiologic and imaging sciences, a society or professional organization supports the individuals holding the registry credential and accreditation agencies govern the educational programs in the specialty professions.

The AHRA (association for medical imaging management) was formed to provide an organization for radiology administrators to share problems and solutions as well as to create continuing education opportunities. To provide further certification, the CRA (certified radiology administrator) examination and credential were created. The CRA examination has been shown to be a valid measure of radiologic and imaging sciences administration knowledge and skills.

The role of the radiology administrator must grow simultaneously with the entire field of radiology, and such growth requires administrators with a variety of management skills. An individual who combines management abilities with technologic expertise is a valuable asset to the radiologist, the radiology department, and the hospital. Such individuals are in demand, and opportunity awaits the radiologic technologist who plans to fill this need.

RADIOLOGIC TECHNOLOGIST EDUCATOR

Roentgen's discovery of x-rays in 1895 established the need for specialists such as the **radiologist** (a physician who specializes in the medical science of x-rays and other radiation energy forms to diagnose and treat disease) and the radiologic technologist. Educators for the radiologists and technologists were needed so that enough people could be trained to enter the field. The need for the educator in Europe was established in France during World War I. During this bloody conflict, the Polish-born scientist Marie Sklodowska Curie (1867–1934) realized that radiologic

units were needed to x-ray the wounded. She designed several "x-ray cars," which were mobile x-ray units available for surgeons and physicians at the front. From 1916 to 1918, Curie trained 150 technicians—the first formally trained x-ray technicians in Europe—to operate these mobile units.

During this same period, formal training began in the United States. Eddy Clarence Jerman (1865–1936) was employed by the Victor X-ray Corporation, and in 1917, he was assigned to develop an educational program for operators of x-ray equipment; this was the beginning of a formal educational program. In 1920, 13 of these trained operators met with Jerman at the Victor X-ray Corporation in Chicago to organize a professional society, which today is known as the ASRT.

With the beginning of formal training in x-ray technology, a means and method for the examination and certification of individuals trained in the profession became necessary. In 1922, the American Registry of X-ray Technicians was established. In 1933, formal training of x-ray technicians was recognized. Over the years, thousands of individuals trained in the art and science of radiography have become registered by the ARRT.

With the dynamic growth of radiology and radiologic technology, the need for educators is greater today than ever before. Hospital certificate programs, associate's degree community college programs, bachelor's degree, and master's degree programs in radiologic technology require the services of educators who are experts in radiologic technology and who are able to communicate this knowledge to the student radiologic technologist. The expertise an individual must bring to the classroom includes not only radiography but also higher educational theories. Today, when educators are held accountable not only by the profession but also by their students, the responsibility of the **radiologic technologist educator** is to enter the classroom with knowledge and experience in both radiologic technology and education.

The radiologic technologist educator must demonstrate competency in curriculum design and program planning. The individual should be able to design a model program, with particular attention given to course outlines, lesson plans, assessment, and use of textbooks and course materials.

The radiologic technologist educator should also take courses in the historic foundations of education and the philosophic and psychological foundations of education. Student advising is very important, and it can demand a great amount of time. A radiologic technologist who is pursuing a degree in education should be competent in educational psychology. Instructional skills can be developed in numerous ways, and many educational programs require that candidates prepare "micro courses" and present them to their peers. Preparing such micro courses is an excellent opportunity for the education major candidate to write objectives for the course, prepare course outlines and lesson plans, and prepare audiovisual aids.

Evaluating and assessment are also important to the educator, because **formative evaluations** (in-depth, individualized assessments of knowledge) and **summative evaluations** (in-depth appraisals of knowledge that result in final grades or a certifying examination) are valuable tools for gauging the progress of class presentations and for determining final grades. Programmatic assessment is crucial to ongoing program effectiveness. Educational programs throughout the country offer courses in interpreting educational research and in methods of item writing that will be important throughout an individual's career.

The science of radiography is becoming more sophisticated and requires high-quality educators. Presenting a background that is indicative of the profession and the educational knowledge and skills to transmit this information to future generations of radiologic technologists is the educator's responsibility.

Many radiologic technologist educators continue their educational pursuit toward doctoral degrees.

Those of us involved in radiography education, as well as education in the other radiologic technology specialties find it extremely fulfilling to prepare the future of our profession.

The qualifications for a full-time program director, didactic program faculty, full-time clinical coordinator, and clinical instructor are addressed in the accreditation standards published by the Joint Review Committee on Education in Radiologic Technology (JRCERT). Program director and clinical coordinator positions require a minimum of a master's degree and baccalaureate degree, respectively.

See Box 16.12 for career information.

CONCLUSION

The growth of radiography since Eddy Jerman and Marie Curie trained x-ray operators has been indicative of a science that is continually striving to serve and protect quality of life. Pursuing the education necessary to keep abreast of professional development is the responsibility of the radiologic technologist.

Several areas for specialization exist in the profession of radiologic technology. Entrance into these areas is usually a matter of the technologist's preference, but other factors

---

BOX 16.12   Radiography Educator Careers

For information on a career as a radiography educator, visit:

Joint Review Committee on Education in Radiologic Technology: www.jrcert.org

Association of Collegiate Educators in Radiologic Technology (ACERT): www.acert.org

Association of Educators in Imaging and Radiologic Sciences (AEIRS): www.aeirs.org

For degree programs specific to radiologic technology or radiologic technology education, use any comprehensive Internet search engine, such as Google (search by topic)

---

may also be included in the decision, such as employment opportunities, educational requirements, and access to educational programs.

Radiologic technologists interested in career mobility have several options for investigation. Regardless of the career pathway, advanced education holds the key to upward as well as lateral mobility. In any case, achievement of goals and graduation is a time of pride and accomplishment (Fig. 16.20).

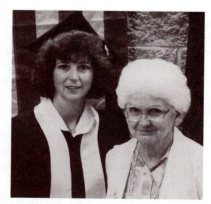

Fig. 16.20 Graduation, the celebration of career advancement and accomplishments.

QUESTIONS FOR DISCUSSION AND CRITICAL THINKING

1. Discuss the breadth of responsibilities required of a radiographer.
2. Enumerate advantages to specializing in radiography.
3. List the five main areas of responsibility in each specialty of radiologic technology.
4. Explain what is meant by practice standards and the scope of practice in the profession.
5. Discuss advantages to working in each of the radiologic technology specialties.

BIBLIOGRAPHY

Adams N. *Forensic imaging technologist: dream job?* Available at http://www.carestream.com; 2019.

American Registry of Radiologic Technologists. Available at http://www.arrt.org; 2019.

American Society of Radiologic Technologists. Available at http://www.asrt.org; 2019.

Association of Collegiate Educators in Radiologic Technology. Available at http://www.acert.org; 2019.

Association of Educators in Imaging and Radiologic Sciences. Available at http://www.aeirs.org; 2019.

Bergonie J, Tribondeau D. *Comp Rend.* 1904; 47:400.

Callaway W. *Mosby's comprehensive review of radiography.* ed 7, St. Louis: Elsevier; 2017.

Harris EL, Young P, McElveny C, et al. *The shadowmakers, a history of radiologic technology.* Albuquerque, NM: American Society of Radiologic Technologists; 1995.

Lampignano J, Kendrick L. *Bontrager's textbook of radiographic positioning and related anatomy.* ed 9, St. Louis: Elsevier; 2018.

Long B, Rollins K, Smith B. *Merrill's atlas of radiographic positioning and procedures.* ed 14, St. Louis: Elsevier; 2020.

GLOSSARY

A

academic course Course of study offered by an accredited postsecondary educational institution such as a college

accreditation Process that a health care institution, provider, or program undergoes to demonstrate compliance with the standards developed by an official agency

adolescent A teenager

affective learning Related to an individual's feelings and emotions such as joy, sadness, evenness, or natural impulses

Affordable Care Act Federal law requiring all citizens to purchase health insurance; has had a mixed effect on health care costs

AHRA: The Association for Medical Imaging Management Professional organization primarily for managers of imaging departments

air kerma Measurement of radiation in-air; unit is the gray (Gya)

algorithms Mathematical formulas used by computers to create digital radiographic image

allied health Group of specialized, professional health care workers; professions resulting from specialization because of advancements in science and technology

American College of Radiology (ACR) Professional organization of physicians that specializes in radiology

American Registry of Radiologic Technologists (ARRT) Professional organization that certifies and registers qualified radiologic technologists

American Society of Radiologic Technologists (ASRT) Professional organization for radiologic technologists

angiogram Radiographic study of arteries and/or veins

angiographer Technologist who engages in radiography of the blood vessels of the body

Anna Bertha Roentgen Wife of Wilhelm Roentgen, discoverer of x-rays; her hand was the first human x-ray image ever produced

anode Electrode toward which negatively charged ions migrate

antiseptics Substances that prevent or retard the growth of microorganisms

arteriogram Radiographic study of the arteries of a particular region of the body

arthrogram Radiographic study of the structures in and around a joint

as low as reasonably achievable (ALARA) Basis for the policies and regulations of the National Council on Radiation Protection and Measurements (NCRP)

Association of Collegiate Educators in Radiologic Technology (ACERT) Professional organization that exists to provide forums for educators to share ideas, strategies, and solutions in their quest for educational excellence in radiologic science

Association of Educators in Imaging and Radiologic Sciences (AEIRS) Professional organization of educators that exists to promote excellence in education and the common goal of safety in the practice of radiologic technology

attention Act of concentrating on one activity to the exclusion of others

attitude Mental position with regard to a fact or state; a feeling or emotion

B

background radiation Radiation from the sun and stars; radioactive elements in the earth; and radioactive substances found in food, water, and air

barium Element used to provide radiographic contrast of gastrointestinal structures

barium enema Radiographic examination of the colon involving the use of a contrast agent

barium platinocyanide Substance which coated the photographic plates used by Roentgen in the discovery of x-rays

Bergonié-Tribondeau, law of Law that states that cells are most sensitive to the effects of ionizing radiation when they are rapidly dividing, immature, and non-specialized

biennial Every 2 years (24 months)

body mechanics Action of the muscles in producing body motion or posture

bone densitometry Uses x-ray energy to measure bone mineral density

C

carcinogenic Substance or agent that causes cancer

cardiac arrest State of complete cessation of the heart's action

cardiopulmonary resuscitation (CPR) Restoration of the function of the heart and lungs after apparent death

career mobility Progress of an individual from one career group to another

carte blanche credits Discretionary credits awarded by an institution of higher learning

case law Law that arises from the interpretation by judges of constitutions, statutes, and administrative regulations; these interpretations are set forth in court opinions, which are the result of the litigation of disputes between two or more parties

category A Continuing education activities that have received approval *before* the activity attendance by a **recognized continuing education evaluation mechanism** (RCEEM).

cathode Filament that gives off electrons when heated

certificate of need (CON) Certificate issued by a review committee to the purchaser or applicant after the need for the equipment or expansion has been established and well-documented

certification Guarantee of qualifications indicated by the issuance of a certificate

child abuse Mistreatment of a child by a parent or guardian, including neglect, beating, and sexual molestation

civil assault Tort that is the result of intentional conduct; occurs when a person has a reasonable fear of physical touch or injury as a result of another person's use or threat of force (e.g., telling a patient in a threatening voice to hold still)

civil battery Tort that is the result of intentional misconduct; occurs when a person intentionally and inappropriately touches another person without consent (i.e., health care professionals treating a patient without that patient's valid consent)

clinical competency evaluation Standard used for evaluating a student's work performance within the clinical laboratory setting; is based on clearly defined levels of expected performance of various essential tasks

cognitive learning Intellectual process by which knowledge is gained through various methods such as books, class work, judgment reasoning, lectures, memory, or perception

collimation Restriction of the primary radiation to a limited area

collimator Device attached to the x-ray tube to reduce the exposure field size to the size of the IR, thus protecting the patient from unwanted radiation

commercial representatives Individuals who work for imaging-related companies in sales or support roles

compliance Agreement with published educational standards and validated by the evaluation process

compliance evaluation Inspection and testing of x-ray units to ensure that their performance is within the mandated and recommended safety standards

Compton scatter Interaction in matter in which the incident photon ejects an electron from its orbit, giving up only part of its energy and resulting in the photon's change in direction with less energy

computed radiography (CR) Process in which an image is created when the x-rays exit the patient and strike a cassette containing an imaging plate

computed tomography (CT) Radiographic cross-sectional electronically created image that uses a very small beam of radiation

computer memory Area of computer where information is stored

confidentiality Policy of maintaining privacy and reliance with entrusted patient information

conflict Tension resulting from disagreements of incompatible inner needs or drives

conflict resolution Act of solving provider-customer problems; the tools of conflict resolution include listening, emphasizing, building trust, and developing solutions; these tools can also be used to solve interdepartmental conflicts

contagious disease Condition that may be contracted by the direct or indirect contact with the pathogen that causes the disease

continuing education credit (CE credit) Unit of measurement for continuing education activities; one credit is based on one 50-minute contact hour

continuing qualifications requirement (CQR) Process used to assess whether technologists' level of knowledge has kept up with changes and advances in the field; begins with a non-graded self-assessment; determines in what areas, if any, prescribed CE activities must be completed. CQR takes place every ten years

contrast media Solutions or gases introduced into the body to provide radiographic contrast between an organ and its surrounding tissue

controlled environment Artificial environment used to verify the results of an experiment

convulsions Violent, involuntary muscular contractions; spasms

creed Set of fundamental beliefs

critical thinking Act of making wise decisions based on a set of universally accepted values

CT (computed tomography) technologist Registered technologist specializing in CT scanning procedures

customer service cycle Patient's entire care experience, including any interaction the patient has with the radiology department

cyclotron Chamber that makes it possible to accelerate particles to high speeds to use as projectiles

cystogram Radiographic study of the bladder

cytotechnologist Health care professional who stains, mounts, and evaluates human cells to determine cellular variations and abnormalities such as cancer and other physiologic changes

D

defendant Individual being sued in a lawsuit

defensive medicine Any waste of resources that is the result of a change in physicians' patterns of practice as a result of the threat of malpractice

density Term often used to describe the dark areas on a radiographic image; in digital imaging, image brightness refers to the amount of light emission from the computer monitor. Areas of greater brightness correspond to less dense areas of the body, while areas of lesser brightness demonstrate denser regions of anatomy

deoxyribonucleic acid (DNA) Genetic material in the nucleus of all cellular organisms

diagnostic medical sonography Diagnosis of a disease process, or the imaging of a certain condition such as pregnancy, by the administration of high-frequency, non-ionizing sound waves

diagnostic medical sonographer Registered technologist specializing in the practice of sonography

diet Daily intake of food and water

dietitian Clinician who applies the principles of nutrition and management in administering institutional food service programs, plans special diets at physicians' requests, and instructs individuals and groups about the application of nutrition principles in the selection of food

digital communications in medicine (DICOM) Computed imaging procedures such as DR, CT, nuclear medicine, digital sonography, and MRI use DICOM as a common language

digital imaging, digital radiography Images generated by a computer in which a numerical value is assigned to a color or shade of gray

digital radiography See digital imaging

dignity State of honor, esteem, or being worthy

direct digital radiography (DR or DDR) Process in which an image is created when the cassette is eliminated and replaced by an imaging plate

disease Disorder of bodily functions; the pattern of response to an injury

disinfectants Substances used to destroy pathogens or render them inert

distortion Misrepresentation of the size or shape of an object on the radiographic image

diversity Condition of being different or having differences

dosimetry Measure of radiation dose to an individual

E

effective dose limit Limit to the amount of radiation that individuals should be exposed to; unit is the sievert (Sv)

effective listening Important tool used in conflict resolution; includes establishing eye contact; using face, voice, and body to express concern; and avoiding interrupting

elder abuse Mistreatment of an older person that may be physical, financial, or psychological

elongation Type of shape distortion where the anatomy is demonstrated longer than it actually is

emancipation Freedom from restraint or influence

emancipatory learning Awareness of the forces that have created the circumstances in one's life and taking action to change them

emergency medical personnel Those who administer basic life-support skills and therapy in emergency situations through radio communication with a physician

emerging infectious disease Condition of an infectious origin whose incidence in humans has either increased within the past two decades or threatens to increase in the near future

emotionality Quality or state of a sound emotional balance

empathy Understanding and acceptance of another person's feelings or experience

epidemic Outbreak or product of sudden rapid growth or development that affects many people at once

erythema dose Dose of radiation that causes the skin to turn red

esophagram Radiographic study of the esophagus

events Steps a patient takes to have a radiologic examination, which include making the appointment, arriving at the hospital, registering, having the examination performed, and being released

excretory urography Radiographic studies of the urinary system

exposure factors Adjustment of the voltage, amperage, distance, time, and other factors considered in the determination of producing a diagnostic radiographic study

external preparation Removing the patient's clothing and jewelry before radiography

F

fainting Sudden fall of blood pressure with a loss of consciousness

false imprisonment Tort resulting from intentional misconduct such as restraining or confining a person without proper authorization or consent

fiber optics Fibers with the unique characteristic of transmitting light

flow chart Chart used by administration personnel to show pathways for routing or sequencing work unit activities; may be used to indicate personnel mobility or positions

fluoroscopic studies Radiographic studies obtained using a fluoroscope

fluoroscopy Procedure using x-rays to image inner parts of the body in movement and motion

fog Any unwanted densities on a radiographic image, such as those caused by scatter radiation

forensic imaging Assists pathologists, and in some cases anthropologists, to identify remains or to verify the cause of death.

foreshortening Type of shape distortion where the anatomy is demonstrated shorter than it actually is

formative evaluations In-depth individualized assessments of knowledge

G

gonad General term that describes both male and female reproductive organs

gravity line Imaginary vertical line that passes through the center of gravity; refers to the center of gravity when a person is in the standing position

gray (Gy) Unit of measurement describing the absorbed dose of radiation in air (Gya) or in tissue (Gyt)

grid Device placed between the image receptor and patient designed to absorb the multidirectional scatter radiation

H

health State of complete physical, mental, and social well-being

health information management (HIM) Personnel whose work encompasses a wide variety of tasks, including planning, organizing, and directing the activities of a health information management department

health maintenance organizations (HMO) For a monthly fee, provide all necessary medical care at no additional charge.

herd instinct Natural cohesiveness within a social group

hierarchy of human needs Arrangement of needs into a graded or valued series, from the most basic to the highly complex

histologic technician Clinician who sections, stains, mounts, and identifies human tissues for microscopic study

hospital information system (HIS) Computer system that combines all relevant information pertaining to operations, patients, and billing

hospital safety committee Representative of a broad scope of activities for developing and monitoring safety in all areas of the hospital, such as electrical systems, sanitation and infection control, waste disposal, and fire and other disaster safety plans

human-made radiation Radiation created by instruments

hysterosalpingogram Radiographic study of the uterus and fallopian tubes

I

image brightness The brightness of the radiographic image is the amount of light emission from the computer monitor. Areas of greater brightness correspond to less dense areas of the body, while areas of lesser brightness demonstrate denser regions of anatomy

image contrast May be defined as the visible difference between two areas of brightness in the displayed image

image intensifier Device that electronically improves and enhances fluoroscopic images and transmits them to a flat-panel monitor

image receptor (IR) Device that absorbs the x-rays exiting the patient

imaging informatics Provides for the efficient management of imaging services, proper patient care, and accurate billing for services.

incidents Steps taken by the radiographer when performing an examination of a patient

independent clinical performance Work that is performed by an individual without supervision, which may involve simple or complex levels of problem solving and decision making relative to completing the task

infant Child during the earliest period of life

in-service education Knowledge, information, and skills related to specific tasks, policies, and procedures provided by the institution

inside customers Patients who come to the radiology department from inside the hospital

institutional accreditation Seeks to assess the overall quality and integrity of an institution.

interaction To act on each other, often with reciprocal influence; may involve verbal and nonverbal communications systems with two or more individuals

internal preparation Use of enemas to cleanse the abdomen to view internal structures radiographically

interventional radiography Subspecialty of special procedures that aids in patient treatment by replacing surgery or complementing the surgical process; certification by the American Registry of Radiologic Technologists

inverse square law Law that states the intensity of radiation is inversely proportional to the square of the distance from the source of radiation.

iodine Element used to provide radiographic contrast between organs and blood vessels

ionizing radiation Radiation having sufficient energy to produce ions (i.e., displace electrons from atoms); x-rays are one form of ionizing radiation

isolation room, isolation unit Place to confine the patient with a disease to protect the patient from microorganisms carried by people entering the room or to protect other patients or people working with the patient

J

Johann Wilhelm Hittorf Conducted experiments with cathode rays, which are streams of electrons emitted from the surface of a cathode.

K

kilovoltage Electrical factor that controls the energy of the x-ray beam; 1000 volts

L

latent period Time between the initial irradiation and occurrence of any biologic change

legal guardian Person who has legal authority to make medical decisions for a child, often a parent

license Agency- or government-granted permission that is issued to an individual to engage in a given occupation on finding that the applicant has attained the degree of competency necessary to ensure that the public health, safety, and welfare are reasonably well-protected

life-cycle cost Acquisition cost of equipment plus the cost of maintaining it through its useful life

long-term memory Memory-storing process requiring organization and association of information

lymphocyte Mature white blood cell

M

magnetic resonance imaging (MRI) Cross-sectional, three-dimensional imaging modality that creates digital images by the use of a strong magnetic field and radio waves instead of radiation

magnification Type of size distortion where the anatomy is demonstrated larger than it actually is

mammogram Radiographic study of the breast

mammography Radiographic examination of the breast requiring the use of specialized equipment

maudlin Tearful, often weakly emotional; effusively or foolishly sentimental; lachrymose

Medicaid Government-provided health insurance for the poor

medical technologist Clinician skilled in chemical laboratory analysis, as well as complex and specialized tests, for the diagnosis and treatment of disease

Medicare Government-provided health insurance for older adults

memory retrieval Recalling, recovering, or obtaining events and experiences stored in memory

memory storage Recording of facts, images, sounds, pleasure, pain, and other life experiences in an individual's memory

microprocessor speed Speed at which a computer can perform calculations

milliamperage Electrical factor that controls the amount of x-rays produced; 1000th of 1 ampere

milliampere-seconds (mAs) Milliamperage multiplied by time; mAs controls the amount of radiation produced in the x-ray tube

mobile unit, portable unit X-ray machine designed for easy movement for radiographing or fluoroscoping patients outside the radiology department (e.g., in surgical department)

modesty Propriety of dress, speech, or conduct

moments of truth Times when a patient forms an opinion concerning the quality of service

morals Principles or rules of right conduct or the distinction between right and wrong

morbidity Occurrence of disease; a diseased state

mortality rate Rate of death from various conditions

MRI technologist Registered technologist who specializes in magnetic resonance imaging scanning and procedures

myelogram Radiographic study of the subarachnoid space of the spinal cord

N

negligence Breach or failure to fulfill a required standard of care, which is determined by the degree of care or skill a reasonable medical professional would have provided under the circumstances

nuclear medicine Diagnosis or treatment of a disease process by the administration of a radioactive material to a patient or patient's specimen

nuclear medicine technologist Registered technologist who specializes in nuclear medicine procedures, operating imaging devices, and injecting radiopharmaceuticals

nuclear radiology Branch of radiology that uses radioactive materials for diagnosis and treatment

nurse Health care professional who provides physical and emotional support a patient; teaches patients and their families about illness and therapy; makes observations and assessments that are useful to other staff members, takes patient histories, gives physical examinations, and administers prescribed treatments.

nursing profession Oldest, largest, and most readily identified of the health professions other than medicine

O

objectivity Quality or state of being able to interpret a situation from an unbiased point of view rather than from one's own subjective view

object-to-image receptor distance Distance from the anatomy being imaged to the image receptor

Occupational Safety and Health Administration (OSHA) Federal agency responsible for establishing safety standards for the workplace; an environmental watch to guard against pollution and waste-disposal hazards

occupational therapist Clinician who evaluates the self-care, work-and-play and leisure tasks, and performance skills of patients with disabilities; plans and implements programs, social activities, and interpersonal activities designed to restore, develop, and maintain the patient's ability to perform activities of daily living

organizational chart Chart depicting established lines of authority, responsibility, and accountability

outside customers Patients who come to the radiology department from outside the hospital

P

PACS administrator Registered technologist who specializes in managing the picture archiving and communication system in radiology

pandemic Disease occurring over a wide geographic area and affecting an exceptionally high proportion of the population

passive participation Listener or observer in a situation who is not physically participating or contributing in any way

pathogen Any virus, microorganism, or other substance that causes disease

patient consent Form signed by the patient giving consent for certain medical situations, such as surgical procedures, research, some medical tests and therapeutic procedures

peer review Characteristic of the program review process conducted by a qualified site visit team and accrediting agency

perceptions Observations, mental images; a result of perceiving

personal obligation Related to an individual's character, conduct, motive, or private affairs, as opposed to obligations expected of an institution or organization

personality Characteristics that define a person's identity as determined by heredity and environment, including personal attitudes, interests, values, and knowledge

personnel monitoring Measuring the radiation exposure received by personnel in the performance of their duties

phantoms Solid or liquid materials whose x-ray attenuation and scattering properties are similar to those of body tissues

photoelectric effect Interaction of a photon in which all its energy is absorbed by an electron, resulting in the ejection of the electron from its orbit

physical therapist Clinician who uses physical agents, as well as biomechanical and neurophysiologic principle and assistive devices, to relieve pain and restore function after disease, injury, or loss of a body part

physician assistant Health care professional who, under the supervision of a physician, performs tasks usually conducted by the physician

picture archiving and communication system (PACS) Computer system that brings digital images together with

radiologist reports and image evaluation; provides for accurate diagnosis, reporting, and billing

plaintiff Person who initiates the lawsuit in a civil case

portable radiography and fluoroscopy See mobile units

position description Synonymous with job description but also connotes a broader scope of activities and defines the place on the organizational chart based on tasks and duties

positioning skills Accuracy with which the patient, part, and x-ray tube are aligned for a given projection

positron emission tomography (PET) Uses a radiopharmaceutical agent to evaluate the physiologic condition or function of an organ or system in the body.

prefix Affix attached to the beginning of a word, base, or phrase to create a word or inflectional form

practice standards Guidelines for safe practice; they provide descriptions of practice criteria, education levels, and the quality of patient care expected.

primal stresses Original, first, or fundamental fight-or-flight response

probation Status that denotes noncompliance with mandated requirements

procedures manual In-house procedures and policy manual designed to meet accreditation standards, state and federal standards, and hospital codes

programmatic accreditation Addresses compliance with accreditation standards at the program level

prospective payment system (PPS) Government's response to the high cost of health care; reimburses hospitals for tests and treatments for patients with Medicare and Medicaid

psychologic care Care received to develop and maintain a healthy balance between rational thoughts and emotions

psychomotor learning Muscular action or practical execution of previously learned material that is believed to come from a conscious mental activity

Q

quality assurance, quality control Quality assurance refers to the total delivery of patient care and service; quality control refers to safety of equipment operation

quality assurance technologist, quality management technologist Registered

technologist who oversees a system of activities whose purpose is to provide assurance that overall quality is being maintained

R

radiation safety committee Group responsible for monitoring and maintaining a radiation-safe environment

radiation therapist Clinician who, under the direction of the radiation oncologist, delivers radiation therapy treatments by exposing specific areas of the patient's body, usually affected by tumors, to prescribed doses of ionizing radiation

radiation therapy Treatment of disease, usually cancer, with ionizing radiation

radioactivity Property of certain elements to emit rays or subatomic particles spontaneously from matter

radiographers Registered technologists who specialize in the field of radiography

radiography curriculum Course of study prepared by the American Society of Radiologic Technologists used in all radiography programs

Radiological Society of North America (RSNA) Professional organization for radiologists

radiologic technologist Health care professional skilled in the theory and practice of the use of radiation in the diagnosis and treatment of diseases and the delivery of quality patient care and service

radiologic technologist educator Registered technologist who specializes in the education of technologists in the various specialties in the profession

radiologist Physician who specializes in the medical science that manages the use of x-rays, radioactive substances, and other forms of radiation energy in the diagnosis and treatment of disease

radiologist assistant (RA) Supplement to radiologists who assists in fluoroscopy, special procedures, patient handling, and other tasks traditionally performed by radiologists

radiology administrator Registered technologist who specializes in the operation and management of the radiology department

radiology information system (RIS) Computer system that combines all patient information and imaging procedures and billing information

recognized continuing education evaluation mechanism (RCEEM) Organization approved to evaluate and give approval to continuing education activities; for example, the ASRT is a RCEEM for most CE courses

registered technologist Technologist who is documented and officially qualified to practice radiologic technology

registration Verification the individual has met all the requirements of the issuing organization

reinforcement behavior Shapes or modifies behavior by rewarding the desired behavior

res ipsa loquitur "The thing speaks for itself"; applies to a situation that suggests that an injury would not have resulted if negligence had not occurred (e.g., leaving a pair of forceps in the patient's abdomen after surgery)

resolution Distinctness with which images of structures are recorded on the image in digital imaging this is referred to as spatial resolution

respiratory therapist, respiratory care practitioner Health care professional who administers respiratory therapy, testing, emergencies, and medication

respondeat superior "Let the master answer"; requires that an employer pay victims for the torts committed by the employees

retakes Common term indicating a repeat of an examination because of inadequate technical quality

root Basis from which a word is derived

rote memorization To learn word by word; to learn by heart or repeat by heart or rote

S

scaled scores Process by which examiners of comparable ability take different versions

scope of practice Describes, delineates, and defines the boundaries of duties and responsibilities of the practicing professional

seizure Attack such as a convulsion

self-discipline Control over emotions and actions

self-study Report prepared by accredited programs following extensive internal evaluation of all aspects of program operation

shock Profound depression of vital functions, with reduced blood volume and pressure

short-term memory Transient, fleeting memory that fades rapidly

sievert (Sv) Unit of radiation measurement used to describe effective dose limits

site visit Visit during which a Joint Review Committee on Education in Radiologic Technology team is charged with verifying that the self-study report is an accurate portrayal of the program's operation and with evaluating the program's compliance with the established educational standards

smoking Lifestyle factor affecting good health

solicitous Full of fears, concerned, anxiously willing; manifesting or expressing solicitude or concern; may seem somewhat exaggerated in expression

source-to-image receptor distance (SID) Distance from the x-ray tube to the anatomy being imaged

spatial resolution May be thought of as the sharpness of the structures in the digital radiographic image.

sphygmomanometer Instrument used to measure blood pressure

standards of conduct Behavior established by custom or law; recognized and approved behavior

sterilization Destruction of all microorganisms in or around an object

stethoscope Instrument used to hear the respiratory and cardiac sounds in the chest or other body areas

stress Physical, chemical, or emotional factor that causes bodily or mental tension

subject contrast The contrast resulting from the variation of structures in the human body

suffix Affix attached to the end of a word, base, or phrase

summative evaluations In-depth appraisals of knowledge resulting in final grades or certifying examination

surgical radiography Imaging procedures conducted in the operating room during surgery

T

Thomas Edison Conducted extensive research in electricity as well as inventing fluoroscopy

torts Civil wrong, as opposed to a criminal wrong, involving a breach of duty or standard of care that results in injury; can be intentional or unintentional

trauma radiography Imaging of injuries caused by accidents or physical violence

troubleshooting Solving problems by thinking of all possible causes and ruling out each individually

U

upper gastrointestinal (GI) series Radiographic study of the upper GI tract

US Department of Health and Human Services Government department with the responsibility for providing health care and other human-needs services to citizens; also manages Medicare and Medicaid programs

V

venogram Radiographic study of the veins in a particular area of the body

voiding cystourethrogram Fluoroscopic exam of the bladder and urethra while patient urinates

vital signs Blood pressure, temperature, pulse, and respiration

W

W. William Crookes Furthered the study of cathode rays and demonstrated that matter was emitted from the cathode with enough energy to rotate a wheel placed within a tube

Wilhelm Conrad Roentgen Physicist and mathematician who discovered x-rays on November 8, 1895

X

x-ray tube Evacuated glass bulb with positive (anode) and negative (cathode) electrodes

INDEX

Note: Page numbers followed by *f* indicate figures, *t* indicate tables, and *b* indicate boxes.

A

Abbreviations
  in inappropriate or unacceptable, 76
  in language of medicine, 72–74
  in organization, 74
  in title, 74
Abdomen, radiographic studies in, 92–93
Academic courses, 141
Acceptance limits, of radiologist, 127–128
Accreditation, 165
  definition of, 5
  maintenance of, 5–6
  standards, of Joint Review Committee on
    Education in Radiologic
    Technology (JRCERT), 5
ACERT. *See* Association of Collegiate
    Educators in Radiologic
    Technology
ACR. *See* American College of Radiology
Acute radiation syndrome, 100
ADC. *See* Analog-to-digital converter
Administrative evaluation, in quality
    assurance, 127
Adolescents, 56, 56*f*
Adults
  middle age, 56–57, 57*f*
  senior citizens, 57–58, 57*f*
  young, 56, 57*f*
AEIRS. *See* Association of Educators in
    Imaging and Radiologic Sciences
Affective learning, 8
Affordable Care Act, 123
Air, as contrast agent, 92
Air-contrast barium enema, 93
Air kerma, 97
ALARA. *See* As low as reasonably
    achievable
Alcohol, specific causes of death, 35
Algorithms, 49, 74
Allied health, 129
American College of Radiology (ACR), 138
American Registry of Radiologic
    Technologists (ARRT), 136–143
  application process in, 139
  Candidate Status Report of, 139
  competency evaluations of, 10–11
  continuing education requirements of, 11
  examination procedures for, 138–140

American Registry of Radiologic
    Technologists (ARRT) *(Continued)*
  competency requirements in, 139
  content categories of, 139
  educational requirements in, 139
  general qualifications in, 138–139
  registry examinations in, 139
  score report on, 139–140
  history of, 138
  organization of, 138
American Society of Radiologic Technologists
    (ASRT), 142, 144–146
  certification by, 3–4
  competency skill evaluation by, 9–11
  education and curriculum standards of,
    6–8
  legislation and, 146
  practice standards for medical imaging and
    radiation therapy and, 146
  socioeconomics and, 146
  state and local affiliates of, 146–147
Analog-to-digital converter (ADC), 74
Anatomically programmed radiography, 74
Anatomically programmed technique, 74
Anode, 74, 78, 80*f*
Antiseptics, 60–61
ARRT. *See* American Registry of Radiologic
    Technologists
Arteriogram (angiogram), 94*f*
Arthrogram, 94
Arthrography, 94
Artifact, 74
As low as reasonably achievable (ALARA),
    97–98
Aseptic techniques, 61–62, 61*f*
ASRT. *See* American Society of Radiologic
    Technologists
Association for Medical Imaging
    Management, 146
Association of Collegiate Educators in
    Radiologic Technology
    (ACERT), 146
Association of Educators in Imaging and
    Radiologic Sciences (AEIRS), 146
Attention, in learning, 19–20
Attitudes, patient, 108–109
Automatic collimation, 74
Automatic exposure control, 74

B

Background beliefs, and critical thinking,
    23–24
Background radiation, 97
Barium, 92
Barium enema, 93
Barium platinocyanide, 45
Beam alignment, 85, 86*f*
Becquerel, Henri, 48–49
Becquerel (Bq), 97
Bergonie and Tribondeau law, 100
Biologic effects, of ionizing radiation
  genetic, 101–102
  short-term, 100
  somatic, 101
Biotechnology, 33
Bit binary digit, 75
Bit depth, 75
Black, causes of death by
    race, 34
Blur effect, 75
Board of Directors, JRCERT, 6
Body mechanics, 59
Bone densitometry, 160, 160*f*, 160*b*
Boyle, Robert, 45
Breach of standard care, 113
Brightness, image, 75
Bucky, 75

C

Carcinogenic effects, of
    radiation, 101
Cardiac arrest, 60
Cardiopulmonary resuscitation (CPR), 59
Career mobility, 150
C-arm, for radiography, 154, 154*f*
Case law, 111
Cassette, 75
Cathode, 75, 78, 80*f*
CDC. *See* Centers for Disease Control and
    Prevention
Cells, sensitivity of, to ionization
    radiation, 54
Center of gravity, in patient transfer, 59
Centers for Disease Control and Prevention
    (CDC), 33
  in isolation techniques, 60